Greetings from
CANCERLAND

Greetings from CANCERLAND

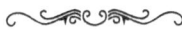

Writing the Journey to Recovery

ALYSA CUMMINGS

iUniverse, Inc.
Bloomington

Greetings from CancerLand
Writing the Journey to Recovery

iUniverse books may be ordered through booksellers or by contacting:

iUniverse
1663 Liberty Drive
Bloomington, IN 47403
www.iuniverse.com
1-800-Authors (1-800-288-4677)

ISBN: 978-1-4759-0987-6 (sc)
ISBN: 978-1-4759-0989-0 (hc)
ISBN: 978-1-4759-0988-3 (ebk)

Library of Congress Control Number: 2012906103

Printed in the United States of America

iUniverse rev. date: 04/10//2012

CONTENTS

Every Ride in the Park

A Country Far Away as Health

INTRODUCTION

Stumbling upon OncoLink, the cancer website for the University of Pennsylvania was a happy accident. An accident because one day in 2002, I did a Google search for cancer poetry, and out of all the hits filling my computer screen, decided to click on www.oncolink.org.

Happy because once I visited OncoLink, I found what I was looking for—poems and survival stories written by real cancer patients. A happy accident, indeed. Ten years later and I know this much is true: when it comes to OncoLink, once I discovered it online, I liked being there so much, I've never left.

Back in 2002, I was a breast cancer survivor relieved to be finally finished with treatment, but still a long way from feeling whole again. Keeping a journal describing my experiences as a cancer patient soothed me. Reading published poems and memoirs written by fellow cancer survivors also moved my recovery forward. But the healing process felt unfinished somehow; I wanted to do more with my journal entries—transform them into poems and more polished pieces. I had begun sharing my writing with fellow survivors in a support group, and based on their positive feedback, I knew that I had more work to do; part of that work was searching for a wider audience.

With some detective work, I connected with Maggie Hampshire by email, shared some CancerLand writing with her, and before long OncoLink began posting my work online. They even gave me an impressive title: OncoLink Poet-in-Residence. Just about every proposed project idea got a green light from my editors: poetry anthologies, book and media reviews, blog entries, poems illustrated with my original photographs.

A relationship with OncoLink helped me find my voice and supplied me with an audience of fellow survivors and clinicians: an empathetic audience that "listened" to my stories and on occasion even responded back by posting encouraging comments. What an amazing, healing connection OncoLink has become in my life!

The poetry and pieces that appear in *Greetings from CancerLand* represent a sampler of my OncoLink writing from 2002-2012. That means that there are highs and lows, moments of celebration as well as those times when bad things seem to happen, one after another. This is not a warning to the reader. Honestly, that's just the reality of cancer treatment. But even as I revisit my CancerLand journey on these printed pages, I am tremendously grateful for my ongoing recovery as well as for my sense of humor that is for the most part, still intact. Overall I must credit the writing; it was the tool and the process that slowly brought me to a healing place.

Why write a book? Why now? Well, it makes perfect sense to me.

I want to add my voice to the literature of cancer survivorship.

I want to hold my CancerLand experiences in my hands and then put them on a shelf.

It's time.

Alysa Cummings
March, 2012

FOREWORD

Monday morning. Open the inbox and there they are staring back at me—100 new emails.

Among them is one from someone named Alysa Cummings.

Like many others, I skim her email and move on, unable to respond in the moment. Too many other issues are competing for my attention right now.

Fortunately, Alysa isn't a sit-back-and-ignore-my-email kind of gal. She persists, emails again and again, until she gets my attention. And so begins a 10 year relationship between the oncology nurses from OncoLink and Alysa, our Poet-in-Residence, friend and colleague.

As oncology nurses, we never headed home from work without feeling the rewards of having made a difference in someone's life. Now as OncoLink editors, a transition to a virtual world of patients has not always been easy; many days we have longed for that connection with a patient or their family. We loved that part of our clinical roles. Alysa, in a way, has filled that void for us.

We have worked with Alysa for 10 years now—communicating mostly through email messages and phone calls—and believe it or not, can count on one hand the number of times either of us have been in the same room with her.

Some might think this "virtual" relationship would be superficial, but that couldn't be further from the truth. Alysa has invited us (along with OncoLink website visitors) to visit with her in CancerLand in a deeply personal way.

We have formed an emotional connection with the person who wrote these stories—in much the same way we did with our patients in our clinical roles as oncology nurses. Over the years, she has made us laugh and cry and we have loved every minute of it.

While it is hard to choose, a few of her pieces stand out as our favorites: *Dear Doctor, Me and My Vampire* and *In the Name of Pinkness*. Alysa has a way of making us relive those moments along with her, making us feel the emotions she felt as a cancer patient in treatment.

At the same time, she has a unique ability to see both sides of the fence. She lets us know (as healthcare professionals), when we are doing something wrong or being insensitive, and she applauds loudly when we get it right.

One of her blog pieces, *It's Not About the Jigsaw Puzzle*, played a role in the design of our cancer center's new radiation waiting area. She put into words what we as nurses instinctively knew; patients benefit from interacting with other patients. We showed her piece to the powers-that-be and reminded them of the importance of cultivating these relationships—to help both patient and caregiver alike.

So, as you can see, our 10 year relationship has been much more than "virtual;" it is a deeply personal, emotional bond that we can't imagine not having. Her contributions to OncoLink are numerous and have given visitors "the softer side" that we, as nurses, can't always relay.

We proudly acknowledge and celebrate her decade as OncoLink's Poet-in-Residence.

Happy Anniversary, Alysa!

Maggie Hampshire, RN, BSN, Managing Editor, OncoLink
Carolyn Vachani, RN, MSN, OncoLink Nurse Educator

YOU ARE HERE

Even when you thought
you were climbing
you had already arrived.
—Erica Jong, "You Are There"

FROM THE MEDICAL RECORD

As
you
recall,
she is
a 45 year old
perimenopausal
white female
who noted a
palpable density
in her right breast
several weeks ago.
Left breast was
mammographically
unremarkable.
There is no
family history
of breast
or ovarian
neoplasia.
She is single
and has no children.
Appears her stated age.
She is alert and comfortable,
in no apparent distress.
Vital signs are stable.
Thank you
for allowing me
to participate
in the care of
this
most
delightful
patient.

Boris

His name is Boris. He is trying to kill me. I won't let him.

And so my CancerLand journal began: with three short sentences, a stream of words that had been swirling around in my head for days. Days that otherwise had been spent in and around the health care delivery system visiting assorted doctors (gynecologist, radiologist, breast surgeon, oncologist) for painful tests followed by frightening results. I remember endless crying jags and repeat phone calls to my insurance company. In my bedroom at night I would stand in front of my full length mirror, my shirt hiked up high on one side, and stare at my upper body—shocked and wide eyed, hypnotized by my reflection, all the while muttering to myself, "so this is what cancer looks like. So this is what cancer feels like."

His name is Boris. He is trying to kill me . . . I repeated these words under my breath like a prayer, my very own disease mantra. Call it the ravings of the recently diagnosed, but the words helped me focus—on the next decision, the next appointment, the next step on the path. The words also kept me slightly sane, all things considered; imagine talking yourself down from the ledge. The words begged to be tapped out on a keyboard, so I followed the urge, liked how it made me feel in the moment and then just kept typing.

I hate Boris. Boris has been lurking in my chest for ten years possibly, hiding, madly multiplying, growing, only now choosing to make his obnoxious presence felt.

Who was Boris? (Yes, I confess that I named my tumor, personifying him as Boris Badunov of Rocky and Bullwinkle cartoon fame).

4

Writing about Boris and plotting his imminent demise helped me wrestle with my first real demon—the fact that I had no control. Never had, never would. Over anything related to cancer, which by definition means life *out* of control.

Boris. Foreign. Evil. Pint-sized. If I can picture my enemy I can fight him; at the very least I can write about him. Am I writing for my life?

I fantasized that I could somehow use my computer to craft a story with an upbeat next chapter or fairy tale happily-ever-after ending. Looking back, that's the only explanation I can come up with, why I felt so compelled to create a record of my day-to-day experiences as a cancer patient. The one thing I *could* control were these words that crowded each other as they quickly appeared on my computer screen; these stories that flowed through my fingertips in such a manic rush; these traumatic adventures that happened to me in a place I began to call CancerLand.

CancerLand: it's this parallel universe, I swear, separate and apart from the rest of life as I once knew it. How did I end up in this wacky Bizarro World filled with freaky language and even stranger rituals?

It was late October, 1998 and I remember being stretched out on my couch in the den watching the evening news. There was one of those predictable stories about Breast Cancer Awareness Month that ended with the reporter promoting monthly self-examination and my hand moved with a mind of its own to my right breast. And that's when I felt it: a lump.

IN THE NAME OF PINKNESS

I'm at the neighborhood Acme, standing in the produce aisle, reaching for some shiny red MacIntosh apples, when I hear a female voice behind me:

Remind all the women in your life to get a mammogram . . .

Startled, I drop the fruit into my shopping cart, look around the store, and try to figure out where the voice is coming from. Suddenly I spot a monitor hanging from the ceiling, right over the potatoes, onions and shelled peanuts. On the screen, an attractive blonde in her mid-thirties is sharing the importance of breast health in a serious voice with a matching expression on her face:

Women over forty should get mammograms every year . . .

Who would argue with her? No one. Not me, certainly. Early detection is key. It's literally lifesaving information that needs to be broadcast to the widest possible audience.

But that day at the Acme, standing in the produce aisle staring up at the monitor, I shake my head and angrily mutter two words under my breath: *enough already!* Thanks to Supermarket TV, I can't even do my food shopping in peace without having to think about breast cancer.

Yes, it's October again. Fall has arrived in rich shades of orange, brown and yellow. Everywhere you look there are signs of the seasons changing: big colorful piles of leaves raked to the curb, mums and pumpkins artfully arranged on the neighbors' front steps.

But in CancerLand this time of year, there's a totally different color scheme. October is the pink month. Truly, madly, deeply pink, everywhere you look: pink ribbons, pink tee shirts, pink hats. Shop online. You can buy pink ribbon stuffed animals, pink ribbon bracelets, pink ribbon shoelaces. On October 1st even Yahoo got involved, looping a virtual pink ribbon around the first letter of their name.

This month there's also dancing, racing, walking and driving for the cure. Go ahead, pick another verb I haven't thought of, and someone else probably already has, and created an event for the cause, all in the name of pinkness. Now, please understand: I have nothing against fundraising, especially if it means we might actually get closer to a cure for cancer in my lifetime. What grates on my nerves is that so much of this well-intentioned effort is jam-packed into the 31 days of October.

Open any newspaper or magazine during the month of October. Odds are there's a human interest story featuring a breast cancer survivor (or two). In these articles, the words *fight, brave* and *battle* will no doubt appear—sometimes in the very same sentence. It makes me more than a little crazy.

On TV, expect the evening news to spotlight a new drug in the War Against Cancer. Or discuss an extremely unappetizing food that you have never heard of before that is now being touted for its anti-cancer properties. Change the channel: Oprah's got Christina Applegate and Nancy Brinker on her show, both crying on camera, at the same time. Seriously, when it comes to Breast Cancer Awareness Month and its insidious pinkness, there's truly nowhere to run, nowhere to hide.

Houston, we have a problem. I'm on October pink overload. And there are a few good reasons why.

Breast Cancer Awareness Month puts a spotlight on breast cancer. (I'm guessing the spotlight is pink, but I could be wrong). That fact by itself is incredibly ironic, because for so many of us on this bumpy road to recovery, breast cancer rarely moves very far from center stage. Survivors these days are strongly encouraged to think of breast cancer as a chronic disease. Which means it's like a hawk flying wide, sleepy circles in the sky high above the earth. To take the metaphor one step further, during the entire month of October, that majestic predator lands, makes a huge nest on my head and squawks loudly non-stop for thirty-one days straight. I'm not kidding. Am I the only breast cancer survivor who feels this way? One thing I know for sure; I don't need an entire month every year to remind me of things I can never, ever forget.

Damn October—the non-stop pinkness, the endless breast self-exam reminders (in the shower, laying down, standing up)—it makes me self-conscious, knocks me totally off balance and shatters whatever "new normal" equilibrium I've managed to build up over time. That's such a shame, because this year should be a time for serious celebration. Let the record show that it's been ten years since my cancer diagnosis. (. . . and I'm feeling more than a little superstitious as I type these words and see them appear on the computer screen. Do I dare plan a Decade in CancerLand Party and risk angering the gods that keep me N.E.D.?)

But when all is said and done, here's the real October demon. Breast Cancer Awareness Month has a way of putting my CancerLand experiences on instant replay. And, unfortunately, all of the intense feelings that go along with this traumatic chapter in my life play back too.

In late October ten years ago, I remember being stretched out on my couch in the den watching the evening news. They were running one of those predictable stories about a breast cancer survivor that ended with the reporter promoting monthly self-examination. My hand moved with a mind of its own to my right breast. And that's when I felt it: a lump.

By Halloween, I was flat on my back on the gynecologist's examination table, staring up at the ceiling while the doctor stuck a syringe in my chest to aspirate fluid from the lump.

I tried to describe that night in my journal:

The holes in the ceiling tiles shift crazily in and out of focus. Dots. Holes. Shadows. Connect the dots. I squeeze the nurse's hand much too tightly and wonder if all the sweat I feel is mine. I smell myself; my own sticky fear. *I don't like it*, the doctor says, finally removing the needle. *It's very bloody. Not acting like a cyst at all.* I sit up and look down at myself. The bandage on my chest is a small square with a bright red circle in the center. *The flag of Japan*, I think to myself. The doctor tries to reassure with lots of nervous pats on my leg. Then the door slams, she's gone and I am alone, cold and shaking all over. I pull on my jeans and trash the paper gown. Something has changed. I know it. Feel it intuitively. For the first time I have seen cancer reflected in a doctor's eyes. I have a feeling it won't be the last . . .

By Thanksgiving I was recovering from my first surgery and being scheduled for a second one because the margins weren't clear. By the eighth day of Hanukkah, I was through my first round of chemo. As thousands of people screamed for the ball to drop in Times Square to welcome the New Year, I watched them on TV and felt the hair on my head release in sections and slide down my back in clumps. Within days I was bald, without an eyelash or eyebrow in sight. All of this happened ten years ago. But when Breast Cancer Awareness Month comes around again, all dressed in pink, I have to stop for a moment and carefully check the year printed on my calendar; it still sometimes feels like it all just happened yesterday.

Maybe my support group buddy Cecelia will be my angel and help me get through Breast Cancer Awareness Month this year. She recently shared a poem she wrote that spoke to me so strongly. "Everywhere I go I carry cancer with me," she wrote. "Now it's not so heavy."

I guess I know what I need to work on before next October.

Dear Doctor,

I am writing to say I'm sorry. I know my apology is almost 11 years overdue, but I mean it. I really do.

With so many doctors on the team working at the imaging center, what are the odds that you would be the one reading my films this year? But as luck would have it, after my yearly mammogram last week, I walked down the hall to chat with the radiologist on call like I always do. And there you were in your long white coat, standing in the semi-darkness peering up at the screens filled with ghostly compressed breast images. No one was more surprised than me.

You must remember me. How could you ever possibly forget the patient who pushed you across the room?

Such an awful day (what I now refer to as the Eve of Diagnosis), and yes, I remember all the details vividly. After reviewing the initial films, you sent me back for more views. Then I had an ultrasound. Next, you stepped into the room and walked over to talk to me.

I don't know, you said, your voice trailing off with uncertainty. *There's something there, but I don't know. I just don't know.* You said those same words over and over again, in a low voice, almost under your breath actually, as if you were talking to yourself, with this incredibly serious expression on your face. But Doctor, I was sitting right there on the edge of the examining table facing you.

Unfortunately I heard you loud and clear.

Maybe there were too many *I-don't-knows* that set me off. I don't know for sure. What I do remember is a metallic taste of panic in my mouth, along with a pounding pain in my head. In the moment there was too much cancer uncertainty for one person to cope with and stay sane. And since I felt so scared, so powerless, so alone and couldn't push away the fear that there was a malignant tumor growing somewhere in my right breast, I did the next best thing.

I put my hands on your shoulders and gave *you* a shove. (an-Elaine-Benes-from-*Seinfeld*-**get-out**-kind-of-shove). I pushed *you* away instead.

Crazy time: in what seemed like slow motion, you stumbled backwards, your eyes wide with surprise. Seconds passed and once you regained your balance, you quickly left the room without saying a word.

Fast forward—one mastectomy, eight rounds of chemo and thirty-five radiation treatments later—and there we were together again last week, face to face. And in that highly charged moment, I couldn't push any words of apology past my lips. I was much too embarrassed. Especially when I noticed that after our eyes met, without missing a beat, you coolly rolled over an office chair to fill the open space between us.

Just in case . . .

THIS BREAST SURGEON

They look at the films together.
Oh, I don't like this. I don't like this one bit, he says.
This breast surgeon points to her x-ray
traces lazy circles with his fingertips,
reaches for a small white writing pad
(the name of a pharmaceutical company
printed across the top);
starts drawing breasts.
He quickly creates a female torso—
just one unbroken line from his black felt tip marker.
A moment later a straight shorter line turns into an arm.
A curved half circle becomes a breast.
Another much smaller circle appears.
Suddenly there's a nipple; then two: a matched set.
In a stupor of silent anxiety, she watches him sketch,
thinks about Picasso;
drawings so evocative
with one simple, continuous line.
And as she spectates, a soothing mantra
spins through her head:
this man has sketched millions of breasts.
He is good at drawing breasts.
He is good at cutting breasts.
He knows breasts.
This breast surgeon.

DIAGNOSIS

His call comes at work; I punch hold and slam
the door shut. *I have bad news. It's cancer.*
One hand that looks vaguely like mine holds the
phone to my ear. The other takes notes on
yellow lined paper. *Cancer.* I write this
word with care, put it in a box. Such a
big idea—little Miss Straight-A student—
I underline it twice,—flash on my need
for a yellow highlighter pen—hear a
voice I think I know beg instead: *give me
something, get me through this day.* "Treatable,"
he says. I press the word into my chest.
"what you've got is treatable," sweet lifeline,
I hold on tight: I twist, I spin, I swing.

CancerLand

For some reason, that's the made-up word I started using to describe my experiences as a cancer survivor: CancerLand.

CancerLand could refer to places like the Chemo Lounge, that room at the end of a long hallway on the fourth floor of the hospital; a place filled with big blue barcaloungers, clicking rapid infusers and blaring televisions hanging from the ceiling.

I was also thinking about CancerLand when I visited a funky shop in the mall named Wig-a-Doo before my hair fell out; a store where the wigs—straight, curly, short, long, blondes, brunettes and redheads—were lined up on shelves with tags displaying each of their names.

CancerLand was the Philadelphia Art Museum on Mother's Day, with hundreds of ladies, all dressed in pink, walking down the steps, into a cheering crowd of caregivers.

And CancerLand was the dark booth at the imaging center, one year after I finished treatment, looking at films with the radiologist, with my heart in my throat until I heard the words, *everything's okay; relax, go get dressed.*

For other survivors, CancerLand might just be the health section at Barnes & Noble, on those three shelves where all the books have *cancer* in the title.

Or a happy day in the waiting room after the final radiation treatment, ringing a shiny brass bell as everybody applauds.

Maybe it's a support group meeting where you and your fellow survivors have a good laugh discussing an article about cancer-sniffing dogs.

CancerLand: it's your life, changed forever now that you've heard the words, "you have cancer." It's a boundary separating who you were before diagnosis and who you might be, right here, right now—physically, emotionally, spiritually.

CancerLand: it's the process of healing and gradually making sense of something veteran survivors call your "new normal." (*Hey, just between you and me, I liked my "old normal" just fine, didn't you?*)

CancerLand. No matter what this make-believe word brings to mind, let's agree that CancerLand is the strangest place you'll ever visit. Good luck making sense of it all.

Like any foreign land, CancerLand has its own crazy lingo and lots of freaky rituals that cancer patients discover as they bump into walls and try to find their way around. Maybe Sylvia Plath was actually describing CancerLand in her poem "Tulips." She wrote, it's "a country far away as health."

THE POWER OF THE PINK RIBBON

There's a ribbon tied in a lopsided bow around a handle on one of my kitchen cabinets. A pink satin ribbon, as a matter of fact.

The pink ribbon arrived by mail on a wintry day five years ago in the first hefty package of information from my insurance company. There it was, peeking out among the forms and pamphlets (*Chemotherapy and You* and *Understanding Breast Cancer Treatment*) for a newly diagnosed cancer patient.

Just a six-inch piece of pink satin ribbon. I picked it up and muttered to myself, *well, look who's a card-carrying member of the sorority now.* Then I remember tying the pink ribbon—my first pink ribbon—in a loopy bow around the nearest brass handle of a kitchen cabinet to keep it away from the two very curious cats in the house.

And there it stayed, through multiple surgeries, rounds of chemotherapy and weeks of radiation treatments, through my lengthy recovery from cancer treatment.

These days, it's quite a conversation starter. When first time visitors walk into my kitchen, they ask, *why is it there? What does it mean?* Some folks are even compelled to comment that this pink ribbon tied in a bow on my kitchen cabinet is starting to look a little tired and droopy. More than a bit bedraggled. Hey, they won't get any argument from me. But this particular cancer relic is staying right where it is. You see, it's part of a cancer ritual.

December will always echo with cancer anniversaries—first surgery, first round of chemo right before Christmas, losing the last of my hair on New Year's Eve. It's hard to forget these passages. Ask any survivor. Such intense experiences can bubble back up to the surface when you least expect them to, even as the years pass. But for me, especially during the last month of the year.

While the rest of humanity rushes around madly buying gifts, (then wrapping fancy paper and ribbons around their purchases), I focus instead on a single pink ribbon that as a symbol helps me make peace with the cancer experience.

I look at this pink ribbon, get quiet and reflect on my life. I think about the painful places where I've been on this long journey back to health. I take pride in all that I have experienced, all that I have overcome. I celebrate my growth and changes, inside and out, as I have moved through healing towards recovery. So here I am—a five-year cancer survivor, ready to cautiously exhale. Such a significant landmark to reach! At least that's what everybody tells me. Yes, I'm still here, with a long list of goals to be checked off my "to-do" list before I'm done.

Let me try and wrap it up nice and neat, with a pink bow. This holiday season, think of me as one extremely grateful lady smiling as she slow dances with N.E.D. The joy I feel is real and it's for the precious gift of remission, for the sweet gift of time. Isn't it amazing how a simple pink ribbon tied in a bow on a kitchen cabinet door can remind me, repeatedly, intensely, vividly, how many different ways the word "present" can resonate?

Seeing Red

A cancer diagnosis. Anger. The cause-effect relationship between a serious health crisis and a person's strong emotional reaction to it seems so obvious. Commonsensical, even.

Maybe that's why my mother wasted so few words on the subject when I went into a screaming "why me" rage over the bad news in my path report. "Get mad. You're entitled," she said, a voice of reason as I melted down in front of her. "Get good and mad and beat this thing."

It would take me a long while to make some peace with my cancer anger. Even longer to focus and do something productive with it. (Truth be told, like anyone in a recovery mode, I need to take anger "one day at a time" and work on it constantly). So while my mother's validation of my feelings felt good for the moment, it did precious little to help me cope with my ongoing rage after diagnosis and through treatment.

Here's one example: I had to get my teeth cleaned before the first round of chemo. Having read my file, the dental tech knew that I had just been diagnosed with breast cancer. As usual, she tapped, poked around and scraped a bit. Like any good patient in the chair, I followed orders to rinse and spit. Halfway through the cleaning, as I reclined under the bright light, with instruments sticking out of my mouth, the dental tech shared this gem of unsolicited medical advice: *If I were you, hon, I'd just get 'em both whacked off.*

Just try to get mad as a sharp instrument probes for plaque below the gumline, while a saliva extractor is wedged beneath your tongue.

Maybe the best you can do is get red in the face and make unpleasant grunting sounds deep in your throat. So I fumed all the way home and once I got there, opened my journal and drafted an angry poem. First I wrote down the dental tech's "get 'em both whacked off" comment and then underneath I wrote;

> *Oh, but she is not me,*
> *and her words are so sharp, so sharp*
> *it feels as if she just has.*

At my request, my dental records were forwarded to another practice. When the office manager asked why I was leaving, I offered to explain the reason why if the dentist would just get in touch. He never called.

And I didn't sit by the phone waiting either, because I had lots of other things to worry about. Namely, getting through multiple surgeries, chemotherapy and radiation treatments that monopolized two years of my life. During that time, lots of other angry pieces landed side by side with that dental tech poem in my cancer journal. Why? Because during cancer treatment, nerve endings can feel like they are sticking out right through your skin: so many injuries, so many losses. It's cumulative and painful, both emotionally and physically. Nothing feels right. Nothing seems good enough. Nothing is the way it should be. Nothing will ever be the way it was before. *And there's nothing that you can do about it!*

. . . except maybe get good and angry. And possibly deal with all that righteous anger by talking it out with a good listener, or by writing it down.

But let's dig a little deeper. What are survivors so angry about? Is it the loss of control? Is it the fist shaking fury of "why me? What did I do to deserve this?" Or could it be some of the little things that start to grate and get on our collective last nerve?

Maybe it's those well-meaning relatives who say the wrong thing at the wrong time, intoning "how aaarrrreee you" with such long faces and pity in their eyes. Maybe we've had it with acquaintances who chatter on and on about their second hand cancer experiences (*Did I ever tell you what happened to my Aunt Rose?*) and don't have a clue that they are speaking in the past tense.

Could we be just a little bit peeved at the tech drawing blood that tries but just can't hit the only good vein left in your arm? Could it be the endless doctors' appointments or the long wait for test results that sets us off? Or have we just had it up to here with all those books and articles that preach the religion of positivity when some days that is a less than reasonable expectation? (*I don't feel like smiling or acting perky*). Or is it that the cancer experience seems more and more like a parallel universe, separate and apart from the life we once knew?

If you are a survivor in CancerLand undergoing or recovering from treatment for your disease, how can you *not* see red?

Really see red then, won't you? Feel the anger flare and burn—in my writing or in the words of another cancer survivor sharing their story of life in CancerLand—and feel our collective energy glowing, red-hot and righteous. Check out the sarcasm. Hear bits of ranting and raving, followed by groaning and grieving. Sense the irony and black humor. It's all there. Tune into it.

To once again quote my mother, when it comes to cancer and anger, we're entitled.

To Hell & Back

The lab technician pats and slaps and stares intently at the crook of my left arm. She presses down purposefully, first in one spot, then another. Her gloved fingers inch bit by bit across the skin on my inner arm, stopping to pat, slap and pat some more. Finally she frowns and shakes her head in frustration. This is my cue to smile sympathetically and ask for her honest professional opinion. "So what do you think? Was I born without veins, or what?"

While my chatter does little to ease the rising tension in the room, I confess I just can't help myself. (*Would an apology help? Make the needle sting a little less?*) "Listen, I'm sorry I'm such a 'tough stick.' But there's got to be a half decent vein in there somewhere, right?"

Still determined to win her over, I smile again and offer up more hollow words of encouragement: "Hey, from what I hear through the grapevine, you're the best. I have a good feeling you'll hit me first time out."

As the old saying goes: if only wishing could make it so.

Unfortunately this scene has played out over the years with so many other lab techs, I know in my heart of hearts, that the odds are stacked against us both. Still this find-my-vein-I-know-you-can patter is quickly becoming a staple in my cancer patient routine. One thing's for sure: pre-admissions testing before surgery is giving my lab tech shtick a major workout; I've run this routine three times today alone.

Why do I bother? Well, when it comes to hospitals, it just makes sense. If you have a needle, scalpel or other sharp object in your hand, I instantly want to be your new best friend. (*Don't hurt me! Please?*) At the very least, let me be more than a disease, more than just another anonymous patient passing through. So I crack bad jokes. And fake bravado I rarely feel. But considering the challenges ahead of me right now as I begin cancer treatment, leading with my personality feels like a reasonable "get along to get through this" strategy.

Bottom line: I am doing the very best that I can, shuffling the lousy cards I've been dealt.

Unfortunately, the bad news is that after four hours straight of pre-admission testing, this Cancer Comedian is not holding up wonderfully well. Cracks are starting to appear in my carefully constructed facade and there might be lots of good reasons why. Maybe I'm sick of roaming hospital hallways not knowing where I'm going. And tired of following colored lines on the floor down and around the bowels of the hospital, gripping my pre-admission test itinerary in my clammy hands like a treasure map (. . . *and once you have received your contrast injection, proceed to room L14 . . .*). Some of today's tests only work on an empty stomach and the fasting has made me feel altered, spacey and disoriented. Then there are the interviews. I have filled out countless forms with the same information and recited the identical medical history to so many strangers in white coats (oncologist, anesthesiologist, physician's assistant) that my head is spinning. I feel the stress slowly building to a critical mass. Still, the reality is that the cancer journey for me has barely begun.

So for right now, I try to focus. Another scan means more directions, more instructions. *Put your clothes in the basket. Tie your gown in the front. Wait here. Go there. Don't breathe. Good. Now breathe.* More burning needle sticks. Dye going in. Lights clicking off and on. Holding still in awkward positions.

If someone would just stop all this hideous "patient processing" for a minute and give me a chance to say something, I just might holler: *Ladies and gentlemen of the healthcare delivery system, I have had more than enough pre-admission testing, thank you very much! Enough already! Please. Stop. Now!*

However, until that fantasy becomes a reality, won't somebody kindly tell me that I've passed my initiation with flying colors? That I'm this close to being accepted into The Club? That in a few more hours, give or take, I'll be an official Card Carrying Cancer Patient in Treatment? That I'm almost there with the finish line in sight? How about a few words of encouragement here? Perhaps in the final analysis, when all the whining is said and done, pre-admission testing has succeeded mostly in getting on my very last nerve.

So here I am, flat on my back, gazing up at a large white circular machine. From this angle, it's just a big metal doughnut to me. In the meantime, the lab technician gamely continues her search for a decent vein in a bruised arm that has already been tapped twice in the same day. Maybe if I focus on the machine I can avoid looking directly at a huge needle with my name on it sitting on a tray. But even out of the corner of my eye, I can see the lab tech and she looks tense. Not confident at all. Maybe that's why I start babbling, ". . . is Tom around? You know Tom from Nuclear Medicine? Nice guy. Soft touch, a touch like an angel, I swear. He found a vein on me early this morning, first time out, no problem and . . ."

But she doesn't call Tom, and in a moment I find out firsthand that my lab tech is definitely *not* the best because she takes a stab at a vein and misses. *It rolled on me. Damn!* (That's right. Go ahead and blame the vein. Bad vein. Bad, bad vein). I breathe in and out, in and out, as she gets ready to stick me again. *I'm really sorry, hon. Hang in there, will you? We have to try at least twice before we go for help.*

This time the tech wriggles the needle under my skin and it hurts so much I suddenly tune into what sounds like a chant with the strangest lyrics: *I'm losing it I'm losing it I'm losing it I'm losing it I'm losing it I'm losing it I'm losing it.* What I'm hearing is my own voice bouncing back at me. In fact I am broadcasting my pre-admissions testing breakdown to anyone who might be listening. And that's exactly what I proceed to do in the next moment: break down, melt down, lose it completely.

The panic attack erupts with a sharp, pounding pain behind my eyes. I wrench my throbbing arm away from the lab tech and howl, like some cornered, wounded animal. *No, no, no, no more, no more.* I shake. I kick. I curse. I roll to my right to jump off the table.

Call it fight or flight. The need to flee is compelling; I'll do anything to get away from her. If I can't run away from my cancer, then putting some space between that hateful needle in her hand and my sore arm right now strikes me as the next best thing.

The darkened control room next door is filled with lots of lady techs busily tracking pale, ghostly images on screens. At the sound of my yelling, they stop pressing buttons and spinning dials on high tech control panels to peer through the tinted glass at me instead. (*Here's the main event of the afternoon, folks; a patient freaking out right before your very eyes*). Three female techs immediately bolt across the room to reach me before I fall off the table. Then three more appear and suddenly there's a crowd, at least seven techs shoulder to shoulder in the suite and one after another they surround the table and throw themselves across me like human blankets. Their combined weight tackles me back onto the table.

Despite the frenzy of activity in the room, no one actually says a word. Quiet moments pass as this panic attack drill team, this circle of women holding me down, works its magic. Their collective body heat spreads deep comfort and soon my tantrum is little more than aftershocks of trembling and lots of congested breathing. I lie there exhausted, beaten up like a boxer gone too many rounds in the ring. Then feelings of intense shame wash over me as I replay mentally what has just happened. And, of course, what has to happen next.

I silently surrender my left arm, extend it willingly. A superstar lab tech (the one they say always hits the tough sticks the first time out) takes me in hand and elegantly hits a vein. Bravo! The dye finally flows where it has to go. I lay back and listen to the whirs and clicks of the big white doughnut shaped machine. *Breathe*, says the mechanical voice. *Hold your breath,* says the mechanical voice. *Breathe*, says the mechanical voice. Now I do my best to follow orders.

When the scan is over, I stumble out of the imaging suite and bump right into my oncologist, Dr. C., standing there in the hallway. "Isn't this a coincidence . . ." He pats the black pager hooked to his belt. "My showing up down here is never an accident. But more importantly, are you feeling any better?" My face turns red. *They paged him. I'm totally mortified.* We walk down the hall together to my last scheduled appointment. All that's left on my list of tests is a simple chest x-ray, but it's a somber reminder of why I'm here today. Dr. C. hovers nearby until it's done.

Despite the fact that it has been many years since my pre-admission testing "incident," the memory of that day played back vividly in my mind like a movie when I read *Close to the Bone: Life Threatening Illness and the Search for Meaning.* In her book, Jungian analyst and clinical professor of psychiatry Dr. Jean Shinoda Bolen, describes eloquently the power of illness to wake us up and jolt us into a new reality.

"Whenever or however that line from health to illness is crossed, we enter this realm of soul. Illness is both soul-shaking and soul-evoking for the patient . . . We lose an innocence, we know vulnerability, we are no longer who we were before this event, and we will never be the same."

For me "soul-shaking" clarity arrived on the heels of one pre-admission test too many; when I got a sharp and bitter taste of what the next chapter of my life would be like, as I left the healthy world and dropped feet first into CancerLand. Other key insights soon followed: I could not control cancer. I could not run away from my condition or wisecrack my way through it either. Still, I desperately wanted to find my way back to whatever my "new normal" would be as a cancer survivor once treatment ended.

According to Dr. Bolen, tuning into such harsh new realities brings a person "close to the bone," and can trigger a transformation, a re-evaluation, a shifting of priorities after deep soul level consideration of "what matters, who matters and what we have been doing with our lives."

Dr. Bolen uses the Greek myth of Persephone, that dramatic story of an innocent taken into the darkness of the underworld, as a way of describing the experience of serious illness, when "the ground gives way under us." *Close to the Bone* goes on to describe the value of myth and poetic metaphor to help us make sense of the intense feelings that arise as we move through sickness towards recovery.

My CancerLand journey had begun . . .

WALKING THE GREEN MILE

The first case of the day has the challenge
of walking the green mile. No gurney. No
wheelchair. Just a friendly stroll pushing an
IV pole down a dark hallway chilled to
subzero temperature. It feels like the
last mile, but there's no electric chair, just
a narrow table. Masks and gloves—MDs
and nurses—a flying saucer of lights
overhead. I enter and all eyes look
my way. How awkward, dramatic even,
this cold, prime time staged scene in the OR.
I feel so compelled to warm up the room,
that I joke, *now that the guest of honor*
is here, I guess this party can begin.

DRAIN RHYMES WITH PAIN

Folks in health care delivery have different ways of letting their patients know that the procedure they are about to perform will hurt them.

In fact, lots of medical personnel I've bumped into over the years are quite creative when it comes to talking about pain. So creative in fact that I'm starting to wonder if they had to take a course called Patient Pain Communication 101 before they earned their CancerLand certification.

There'll be a pinch, they sometimes caution, syringe in hand.

You'll feel a little prick. (Okay, now you're just messing with me and I'm going to laugh out loud . . .)

Then there are the ones who count—approaching patients with sharp objects as they recite: *(1-2-3-ouch!)*

I've also been treated by professionals who hem and haw, but just can't commit: *this* might *sting*, they say, *but just a bit*. Make up your mind!

But I'm most fond of the medical poets I've met who offer up glorious similes—*This won't hurt* too *much*, they say, *just like a mild labor pain*. Women reading that last sentence might be asking themselves a question right about now: how could those three words (mild labor pain) possibly stand side by side in the same sentence? Oxymoron alert!

In CancerLand, no matter how creatively doctors and nurses handle pain-speak, there's typically a postscript. Here's the caveat I hear a lot: *But, you know, everybody's different . . .*

Wait a minute. If everybody's different, does that mean it will hurt me more? Or less? I don't have a clue.

Maybe that's why I remember my breast surgeon so fondly. During my second post-op visit to his office, he grabbed the drain tube snaking out from the incision under my arm with both hands. (*Oh no, was he going to rip it right out of me? Just like that? Right here? Right now?*) My heart started racing; I suddenly felt sweaty and anxious.

From my vantage point—half naked, flat on my back on the examining table—I could only imagine a one-sided game of tug of war that would end badly. With me as the clear loser, hurting, bleeding. After all, he had explained to me that the drain was securely stitched in place.

I waited for some sort of warning from the doctor. Isn't that what they always do? Get you ready for the worst? Help you prepare for the pain? I couldn't believe what I heard next.

This will hurt like hell, the breast surgeon said. *Take a deep breath.*

No euphemisms. No disclaimers. No word play—just a clear warning. What a guy! And a moment later, he proved to be a man of his word. The pain was intense, but short lived. I left the office smiling, one drain lighter, respecting a doc who could speak the truth in simple language that any patient could understand.

But there's a downside. The breast surgeon has graciously offered to "follow" my remaining breast. (Just picture that—where exactly is my breast "going?") So here's my dilemma.

No matter how much I like Dr. M. as a person and respect him as a professional, no matter how grateful I am that he is my doctor, unfortunately I will always associate him with drains and pain and, of course, breast cancer. And isn't that a shame?

QUESTIONS ABOUT CHEMO

The morning I was scheduled to receive my first round of chemo, one of the oncology nurses handed me a hefty folder of information, the words *Chemotherapy: What to Expect* printed in royal blue ink across the front.

Like a straight-A student reviewing notes before the big test, I was immediately drawn to the section describing possible side effects. Minutes passed. The nurse must have noticed the deer-in-the-headlights expression on my face because she patted my arm and said in a soothing voice, "Of course, every patient's different . . ."

I continued to scan the list of chemo side effects and felt my anxiety building exponentially with each new bullet on the page. But then the logical part of my brain kicked in for a moment. I suddenly had questions: lots and lots of questions:

How could drugs make you so sick that you could experience both constipation *and* diarrhea? (*Aren't those opposites? That makes no sense!*)

Patients could run a fever, I read. You might feel chills and experience numbness in your extremities. (*Was this an either/or situation? Or did both hit you at the same time? See previous question*).

Chemotherapy could bring on feelings of fatigue, I read. Or leave a patient in a state of sleepless hyperactivity. (*What the hell?*) I might get nauseous and be repulsed by my favorite foods. I might have strange cravings and gain weight. (*Whaaaaat?*)

Maybe it was the panic talking, but I looked up at the nurse and cracked my very first Bad Cancer Joke. (*It would not be the last . . .*)

"Didn't they forget to mention some of the other side effects of chemotherapy?" I asked sarcastically. "What about locusts, boils and death of the firstborn? And when exactly does my ass fall off?"

Funny, the nurse didn't crack a smile. (Maybe she wasn't familiar with the movie *The Ten Commandments* or the Old Testament).

I waited for a reaction. The nurse still wasn't laughing. But then again, neither was I.

Isn't it interesting how sometimes humor is the coping strategy of choice, especially in those moments when the harsh reality of a situation is just too much to bear?

All these years later, and I'm thinking about that vivid CancerLand moment before I headed down the hall for my first scheduled visit to the Chemo Lounge. It's so obvious that patients in a health crisis need to receive information that is clear and helpful, sensitively written and practical in nature. Using those criteria, my chemotherapy packet failed miserably. End of chemo rant.

MAGICAL THINKING

I was thinking as small children think, as if my
thoughts or wishes had the power to reverse the
narrative, change the outcome.

—Joan Didion, *The Year of Magical Thinking*

If you're a cancer survivor like me, you just might be as guilty of it as I once was.

Guilty of magical thinking, that is.

I remember the first time it happened to me; I had been in CancerLand for a few weeks. The initial shock of the words *I'm sorry, you have cancer* had started wearing off, but ever so slightly.

Trust me on that one.

Slowly but surely I was taking baby steps toward my post-diagnosis "new normal." Case in point: I could actually carry on a civil conversation with someone without crying my eyes out. This was no small feat. And let the record show that I was eating and sleeping normally again, showing up for work every morning and paying my bills on time. All things considered, we're talking fairly high-functional here! At least, that was my goal.

But beneath the carefully constructed I-don't need-any-help, I've-got-everything-under-control façade, I was such a mess. Not in my right mind at all—obsessing over details, crafting lengthy to-do lists, torturing myself with questions that had no simple answers.

My most disturbing feelings, (*who can possibly understand what I'm going through?*) found a home in the privacy of my journal:

> *I have cancer?*
> *No, that's just not possible!*
> *Could the lab have made a terrible mistake?*

Disturbing, indeed. While "Good Patient Me" was busy getting to doctors' appointments on time, taking careful notes and undergoing pre-op tests, one after another, "The Real Me" wasn't completely convinced. My thoughts were twisted and tangled around medical conspiracy theories—wondering if my biopsy slides had been misread, speculating that my file had somehow been switched with somebody else's.

The reality of my medical condition was too disturbing. I couldn't conceive of the words *cancer* and *me* even being in the same sentence. How could I possibly make sense of some nasty new reality that involved cancer cells madly multiplying in my right breast and migrating to lymph nodes in my armpit?

The short answer is this: I couldn't. Not right away. So I found a way to cope. Call it magical thinking, because that's exactly what it was.

Along with stage two breast cancer, I was suffering from a major case of magical thinking. Denial, delusion, and low trust levels blended well with anger of the "why me?" variety. And the magic lingered (*could the lab have made a terrible mistake?*) until I was good and ready to step up to reality, as harsh as it was.

Could it be catching? I think so, because in CancerLand these days, there's spring in the air and lots of magical thinking too. My working theory is that it might show up any place where cancer survivors congregate. Last month, during a conversation with a friend undergoing treatment, magical thinking appeared, without warning or fanfare.

J. and I were chatting on the phone about chemo. We had just discovered what really good friends we were: we had ACT in common. I checked the calendar, counted the days off on my fingers and asked her if she was thinking about getting a wig anytime soon. By my best estimate, she would be losing her hair by the weekend.

"A wig? I don't know . . . ," she began and her voice trailed off. I jumped right in, the voice of experience.

"Well, there are hats, scarves and turbans. They work pretty well, especially when the weather gets warmer," I said. "But I remember how uncomfortable my wig was during the summer, so I ended up wearing a baseball cap most of the time."

"Uh huh . . . ," she said.

Clearly she didn't want to talk about it, but isn't that what CancerLand friends are for? I hoped that I could share a lesson with her that I had learned the hard way.

"Lots of people decide to shave their heads once the shedding starts. You know, take control of the situation instead of losing your hair, bit by bit, day after day until you're bald," I said. "I wish someone had talked me into doing that after my first round of chemotherapy."

The silence lingered. Uncomfortably so. Finally I blurted out the obvious.

"J., forgive me for saying this, but are you thinking that you'll be the only cancer patient on ACT whose hair *doesn't* fall out?"

My hair will fall out?
No, that's just not possible . . .

36

Here's what I believe when it comes to magical thinking. Whether it's me not accepting that my cancer diagnosis is real, even in the face of overwhelming clinical evidence to the contrary . . .

Or it's my friend J. stubbornly hanging onto every hair on her head, imagining that her will is stronger than Adriamycin . . .

Or it's the radiation patient halfway through treatment who says, "I just don't understand why I feel so tired," even though fatigue is the first side effect the doctor described during the initial Radiation Oncology appointment . . .

Or it's the bladder cancer survivor six weeks post-op who offers to help a relative dig up the front lawn to replace a bad sewer line, even though his surgeon has seriously restricted his physical activity . . .

Or it's me, the day I got a mastectomy and insisted on walking the hospital hallways, every hour on the hour.

Here's an excerpt from my journal from that day, that painful moment in time that I tried to distance myself from, by writing about it in the third person as an unnamed 'she':

She walks. Past the nurse's station, the elevator and the family TV room. She walks the fourth floor, pushing the IV pole with her left arm, a miniature pillow clutched against her bandaged right side. She walks. Past her room. Past the open doorways of the other patients. Around again. Another circuit. Moving one foot in front of the other. Walking hurts less than lying down. Feels more productive anyway. Incredibly lifelike. Walking feels like healing. Upright. Moving forward. One step at a time, one foot in front of the other. She walks. Five hours out of surgery and she's upright and clocking indoor hospital miles. What must the other cancer patients in their beds be thinking as they glance away from their TV sets momentarily and see this lady with a denim hat on her mostly bald head walking so slowly, so tentatively, around and around the fourth floor, over and over again? Hey, she's not so sick, that lady doing all that walking, they must be thinking. Look at her. She's okay. She's walking . . .

Magical thinking. Not a bad choice, actually. Quite an appealing alternative in fact, when confronting the reality of surgery, toxic drugs and painful treatments, don't you think? (*Which door would you open?*) Yes, during the most trying times in CancerLand, magical thinking has much to recommend it.

Maybe it's part of the process of hanging onto who we are when cancer threatens to take our identities away. Maybe it's a deep-seated wish for normalcy—that healthy time, before cancer, when we were whole, when we had all of our parts, (they were disease-free and all worked just fine, thank you very much). Maybe it's an attempt to control the uncontrollable. Maybe it's a short course called Coping in CancerLand 101. Maybe it's all that and more.

All this thinking about magical thinking reminds me of a toy I bought years ago at the neighborhood Dollar Store; in fact, it's sitting on the top shelf of my desk; I can see it as I type these words on my laptop.

It's a magic wand—clear plastic, about twelve inches long with a shiny star at the top—the ultimate accessory for a little girl dressing up like a princess. Or relic for a middle-aged breast cancer survivor. The magic wand sits on the shelf over my desk and day after day reminds me of the power of magical thinking to get cancer survivors through crisis to a healing place. (when it comes to symbols, a magic wand just works for me). But, you know what? In CancerLand, I'll take whatever kind of magic I can get my hands on.

CANCER CAT

Hair does not *fall* out. Not really. It's more
of a shedding actually. Dark strands
slip out, sneak free and slide south to nest in
piles at your feet, tickling an ankle on
the way down. I am a cat, a cancer
cat, losing fur as I preen and shake—black
hairs spill across the floor, swirl in corners,
clog drains, coal black clumps thick with soap bubbles.
Baby pink scalp peeks out among the few
strands left—then the cat is gone. In the glass
a pale pasty-faced Shoah babe stares back.
Shave it off. Wear the wig. Get on with it.
All good advice that I choose to ignore;
bewitched by this bald head in the mirror.

CURIOUSER AND CURIOUSER

I walk down the street.
There is a deep hole in the sidewalk.
I fall in.
I am lost . . . I am helpless.
It isn't my fault.
It takes forever to find a way out.
—Portia Nelson, "Autobiography in Five Short Chapters"

I learn by going where I have to go.
—Theodore Roethke, "The Waking"

Survivor's Guide to Post-Operative Body Image

if the
scars
upset
you
that
much
she said,
just stop
looking
at them.
you can
take a
shower
without
looking
down.
yes
you
can.

Cancer Scripts

The therapist listens. Listens to all of it. Listens and nods in places. Murmurs the occasional *uh-huh* to keep me talking. With her encouragement, I slowly spill details from my cancer story. The current chapter just happens to be, Post-Surgery One and Pre-Round Two of Chemo."

I feel the therapist's gaze as I ramble on. Feel her kind grey eyes reading me. Then I sense her focus slowly drift away from my face, up, above my forehead, to stop at an invisible point right above my head. Self-consciously I reach for a handful of hair trailing down the nape of my neck to jerk the wig back into place.

Damn this wig. This long, dark brown synthetic wig named Jennifer. Named no doubt to distinguish her from wigs called Candy (curly brunette), Jasmine (blonde and straight) or Danielle (wavy red). But with wigs having names, I can sit here in therapy as a newbie cancer survivor and actually whine, "I hate Jennifer. She's itchy and uncomfortable. Plus, she makes me look like a female impersonator, don't you think?" Somehow, in this small room, tastefully decorated in rich dark wood paneling and flowery chintz slipcovers, I can openly share my worst here-and-now fear with a trained professional: my nightmare that one day at work, Jennifer will take a nose dive right off my head, leaving me standing speechless and humiliated, (not to mention totally bald), in front of an audience full of strangers.

Bottom line, I am trying therapy on for size. To see how it fits. There's no question I need some help. Cancer treatment is wreaking predictable havoc—from the inside out, from the outside in—on my body, my spirit, my life. What's most upsetting is that when I look in the mirror I can't find any "me" that even looks vaguely familiar.

Springsteen's sad song lyrics are starting to make frightening sense: *I am "unrecognizable to myself."* Maybe cancer has actually changed me into some stranger named Jennifer. Maybe therapy will help me understand this new, disturbing sense of self. Maybe I am trying to put up a good front, playing the part of Super Cancer Patient, but in reality I am slowly losing it. Maybe, just maybe, arm wrestling with appearance demons is a smokescreen for the real life and death issues I am unwilling (or unable) to think about right now. Maybe I don't have a clue.

When our first fifty minute hour comes to an end, the therapist rises from her chair with tears welling up in her eyes and walks the few steps across the room, from her chair to mine, with her arms opened wide. She draws me into an embrace and hugs me uncomfortably close. Releasing me with a warm pat on the back, she says somberly, "It's not just your cancer. You are part of the community of women who live on this planet. We suffer as you suffer. Fight hard. Fight well. We fight side by side with you."

She sends me out the door with a clear and compelling mission: to go off and fight the Cancer Wars for the Good of Womankind. And maybe because that's such a tall order, such a major agenda item on anyone's "to-do" list, I never make another appointment to see her again. Either that, or I don't need to. After all, I have been given my marching orders for this particularly challenging mission: I am Warrior Woman and cancer is the enemy I have to beat to a pulp. Looking back, almost six years after the fact, I know that the "cancer script" the therapist handed over that day in her office played itself out, one scene after another, all the way through treatment.

Truth be told, I put so much energy into playing a role, "courageously fighting the good fight," that Sandy, my favorite oncology nurse, made a comment during one of my last chemo infusions that I will never forget. "Ease up on yourself a little bit, why don't you," she said, "you know, when this is all over, no medals will be given out."

She was so right. When my treatment finally ended, in fact there were no awards for bravery; there wasn't a medal or ribbon or shiny gold star in sight. But maybe it's just as well. You see, because after cancer treatment—the toxic drugs, the repeat surgeries, the radiation—I didn't have much of a chest left to pin them onto anyway.

SYMMETRY IN THE BLUE DRESS

The blue dress hangs in the closet on a
padded hanger, under plastic to keep
the shoulders round. It's a sweater dress with
buttons down the front, a deep vee neck style.
Such a wonderful dress—deep navy blue,
embraces the body in the warmest
wool hug. Rich. Elegant. Timeless. Classy.
The blue dress hangs in the closet and mocks
me as a relic of who I was and
what my body used to look like. Before.
Such a simple dream actually. Me
in the blue dress standing in front of the
mirror, fooling the onlooker with my
cosmetic sleight of hand: both sides matching.

Not Helpful

The late, great Art Linkletter coined the phrase, *Kids Say the Darndest Things* to describe the uncensored and often extremely funny comments young children make.

I'd like to borrow those famous words and edit them ever so slightly to read, *People Say the Darndest Things to Cancer Survivors.*

Why? Because they do. Constantly. If you spend any time at all in CancerLand, you know exactly what I mean.

Words can be hurtful. Especially when you are in treatment: not looking or feeling "at your best." That's when these encounters seem to happen—when you least expect it and aren't strong enough (or in the mood, quite frankly), to handle a verbal assault, unintentional or otherwise.

Maybe it's a relative who cross-examines you for details about your tumor, ultimately asking the painful question, "all that time, didn't you *feel* it?" (How that for a nice dose of blame to totally make your day?)

Or a colleague—like the woman at work who scrutinized my boobs before my scheduled mastectomy, with a quick look down, then left to right and back again, before uttering these memorable words: *well, it's a real blessing that you're so small, now isn't it?* As if the size of a body part has anything to do with how traumatic it is to have it surgically removed.

Or a yoga teacher—like the one who stepped up behind me in class to adjust my warrior pose before she whispered softly in my ear, "no one would ever look at you and guess that you have cancer." Hateful thoughts immediately began running through my head, angry comments that I would never dare say out loud: (*Really? Can I pass as a totally healthy? Have I camouflaged all my scars that well? Do I fool everybody? Good for me!*)

Possibly a neighbor spots you outside on a warm day wearing only a baseball cap to cover your newly bald head, and walks up to boldly ask, *What kind of cancer do you have? What kind of chemotherapy are you on?*

Yikes! I can't make this stuff up.

How do you defend yourself when people violate boundaries this way? What do you say when the angry words, *actually it's none of your business* are right there, on the tip of your tongue? Especially when the conversation turns to a discussion of *God's will*, followed by a reference to the statistical probability of anyone not currently in treatment for cancer being hit by a bus.

Maybe I have to stop and ask myself:

Was I guilty of this sort of rudeness *before* I was diagnosed and knew any better?

Possibly . . .

Is there anything cancer survivors can say or do to protect ourselves?

Absolutely . . .

After a few too many painful cancer-related conversations with various members of the healthy world, I began to interrupt when

I sensed things starting to go badly. Sometimes I put my hand up and did a fine imitation of a school crossing guard stopping traffic. Then I said the following words: *Not helpful. What you've just said to me is not helpful.* At that point, I just walked away. Or in the case of a phone call, I hung up with as much grace as I could manage in the moment. Either way, the conversation was over, I could exhale and focus my energies elsewhere.

You know what? More often than not, it worked.

A CancerLand Holiday Wishlist ... or Please Help Me Get Through the Season

Holidays can be happy, happy, merry, merry, or holidays can get on your last nerve.

You know what I mean? Honestly, it's true. And trust me, cancer may have very little to do with it.

The season that starts with Thanksgiving and climaxes with New Year's Day can drain *anyone* dry, even if you're in the best of health.

The flurry of activity—too many plans and not enough time to do them all. Overeating. Over-spending. Overdoing the celebration. (Did I mention relatives who occasionally overstay their welcome?) It can all be exhausting whether or not you live in CancerLand.

So what can you do for a friend, family member or loved one who's just not "at their best" this holiday season because they are recovering from cancer treatment? How can you help them get through November, December and January and keep a smile on their faces?

After giving this some thought, and checking in with some of my fellow survivors, here's a short wishlist from CancerLand:

Help me feel normal

I'm still me! Sure I've been through some unpleasant medical treatment, and I might not look exactly the same, but I don't want to be treated any differently. And, trust me, I will have zero tolerance for long faces, pitiful expressions and endless "howwww arrrrrre you's" all through dinner.

Help me feel special

Hug me. Kiss me. (Cancer is not contagious). Celebrate with me. Whatever you do, please don't avoid me. I'm grateful to be here—right here, right now—partying with all of you. Keep the invitations coming. Let me join in the merriment if I can, to the best of my ability. The spirit is willing! Let me work out the details.

Help me feel pretty

Losing my hair (along with selected body parts) doesn't mean that I've lost my vanity. If the thought of buying me a gift makes you feel a little bit uncomfortable, (is this the right size? is this the right gift?) do the next best thing: give cash. Love that! Or a generous gift card to one of my favorite stores. I will be eternally grateful and I promise that I'll treat myself to something sacredly selfish and special—all the while thinking lovingly of you.

Help me feel loved

I wish I had a dollar for every time someone said, "Please let me know if there's anything that I can do . . ." Well-intentioned, no doubt, but an actual, caring gesture speaks volumes. The champion crocheter who creates a beautiful afghan that matches my living room color scheme and keeps me cozy during afternoon naps deserves a prize for Best Gift Ever. Ditto for the foodie who drops off a casserole dish filled with gourmet noodle kugel. I can eat some now and freeze the rest for future comfort food attacks. Thank you just doesn't cover it! The neighbor who knows I need help dragging in those garbage cans every Friday morning and just does it without fanfare. That's a real gift from the heart if you ask me. The friend who calls once a week "just to talk," but instead ends up listening. The gift of Beanie Baby miniature stuffed animals—all different types of cats—that keep me company while I'm seated in the Chemo Lounge. Blessings, blessings, all.

Happy Holidays!

Six Month Check-up

My six month check-up is almost over. And so far it's been business as usual. I've been weighed and measured. A nurse has checked my blood pressure. We've been through the "are-there-any-lumps-bumps-or-bruises?" routine. (Classic cancer exam questions. All asked and answered. Check). The doctor has also finished his dance of the fingertips across the lymph nodes on my neck. A six month check-up means getting stuck for blood, means warm hands pressing down, means poking around, means an intense search up and down, for signs of "the enemy" above or below the waist. My six month check-up is almost over. Now maybe my heart can stop its panicky racing and slow down, maybe sound somewhat closer to normal. Not that there's anything normal about being treated by an oncologist. I'm nervous for days beforehand. I'm jumpy once I step off the elevator on the fourth floor of the hospital. So right about now I'm ready to exhale already. I want to get dressed. I want to be somewhere else. (*anywhere* else, to tell you the truth). My six month check-up is almost over. The oncologist washes his hands at the sink, his back to me as I sit on the examining table holding the edges of the salmon colored gown together over my bare chest. I hear the doctor's voice over the splashing sounds of the water as he soaps up, *Everything looks good*, he says, reaching for a paper towel. *In fact, your blood counts are high enough for you to get chemo today.* And with that one simple sentence, I am a survivor sucked back in time, from this reality into another, from here and now back to there and then, to this same room, this same scene years and years and years ago, when a baby blue barcalounger in the Chemo Lounge down the hall was in fact the next stop after the check-up. A primal sound, *nooooooooooooooooooooooo* works its way out of my throat. That's when the onco-doc smiles at the onco-joke he's just played on me.

54

Radiation Crazy Time

Radiation. (a.k.a. crazy time). I thought I had forgotten those seven weeks. But when I least expect it, radiation memories play back in my head like a rerun of some bad Lifetime movie. I can't help myself; I dig out my journal from way back when, read and reminisce about my CancerLand adventures during radiation:

I walk into the basement of the hospital and open the door marked Radiation Oncology. Inside the small room, chairs line the walls and desperately ill people fill the chairs. I sign in and take a seat, since I am now one of them.

I people watch for a bit when I get tired of memorizing the patterns in the rug.

Within minutes, I learn my first euphemism: *treatment.* That's the word of choice. No one here ever says the "r" word: radiation. Just like no one ever says the "c" word: cancer.

How weird is that? Am I the only one who notices this on Day One?

Note to self: bring a book tomorrow. Might be the only way to get through this and stay sane.

Here's what I've learned so far. After the simulation is done, the staff shoots a Polaroid portrait that goes in each patient's file. This helps them pick out each patient from the crowd in the waiting room. Names become irrelevant. Nicknames take their place. One of the techs tells me mine; I am Black-Baseball-Cap-Who-Reads.

Seriously.

One of the nurses tries to make friends with me. She is perky and outgoing. Everything I am not right now. I hate her on sight. Then she starts talking to me and I hate her even more.

You sure like to read a lot, don't you? she says.

You sure are perky and outgoing and obnoxious, aren't you? (Okay, I think these ugly thoughts, but manage to keep my big mouth shut).

Instead I make my infamous 'huh' noise to acknowledge her comment; nothing more. I don't feel very sociable these days, to tell you the truth. So I keep my head down and keep turning the pages in my book.

How rude am I, ignoring her so completely? Where are my manners? Where did they go?

But in my own defense, doesn't my body language scream, **leave me alone**? What is she, blind? Stupid? Both?

In my chemo-addled, over-anesthetized, radiation-toasted body, here's my truth; if you don't acknowledge me, then maybe I'm not really here at all. Blending into the woodwork, flying under the radar, pretending to be invisible feels like the right way to get through radiation treatment.

But the perky and outgoing nurse doesn't give up on me quite that easily. The next day she lifts the brim of my baseball cap, beams me a toothy smile and says, *your hair sure is starting to grow back, isn't it? I feel some fuzz under there.*

Really?

What I feel is a red-hot surge of anger building in me and I need to take a deep breath or two to keep from hitting her. Get your hands off me, lady! Again, I bite my tongue and say nothing. But I do believe that I could strangle the breath out of her and get off in a court of law. I could plead insanity or self-defense. Or both.

Could someone please explain to me how all these other patients are pulling off pleasant, pulling off cordial, pulling off normal social interaction as they go through radiation treatment?

What has happened to me?

COMPLICATIONS

Five weeks after my discharge from the hospital, I am in my breast surgeon's office for a post-op visit following lat flap surgery. The breast reconstruction was done at a hospital in a neighboring state and he has kindly agreed to check the incision for the plastic surgeon.

"How was it?" Dr. M asks gently. "How do you feel? Tell me about it."

"It was horrible," I begin. "Truly hideous." I pause and wonder what else I should tell him.

"Try to talk about it," he says, drawing me out. "Tell me what it was like in the hospital. You know, I did my residency there a long time ago."

I hear myself say the words out loud for the first time: "I felt like a prisoner of war."

"Hmmmm . . ." Dr. M says, nodding his head thoughtfully. "A prisoner of war. Interesting. In a way, I guess you were."

"There were complications," I continue. "Lots of them. Eight days of complications, to be exact. I kept a journal and filled it with all of my complications. It gave me something to do, writing about how horrible it was."

Complications. I have learned that this is the umbrella word health care professionals use to describe bad stuff that happens in hospitals.

Infection is post-op complication number 1.

What kind of infection? Hard to say. But serious enough that they order IV antibiotics the very first night. (I am such an innocent that I conjure an image in my head of the two residents I met right before surgery with dirt lodged under their fingernails). During one of the many brief post-op visits to my bedside, I ask Dr. B, the plastic surgeon, about the source of the infection. "Dr. B., help me understand something. If I have such a serious infection, why do so many nurses and residents keep poking at my incision without wearing any gloves?"

"It's an infection from the inside out, not the outside in," Dr. B says, in a tone reserved for pre-school children and the infirm. "Statistically, this is not an uncommon occurrence after a surgery of this magnitude." What an education I'm getting as I travel in the healthcare delivery system.

Blown Intravenous Syndrome is complication number 2.

On day three in the hospital, my arm begins to swell around the site of the intravenous line. I stop looking at the redness, as if ignoring it will make it disappear. After all, they can only use my left arm, (the axillary dissection was done on the right side), and the line that is going bad is in the best vein I have. Not good. Before long, the night nurse has to pull the IV. I beg for drugs by mouth to fight the infection rather than getting stuck again; that strategy works for a day.

Then it's time to start a new IV. The nurse who's a local legend, infamous for "hitting the tough sticks" (*Kelly's the best. Kelly never misses. We'll get Kelly*), fails to tap anything on the back of my left hand. Ever the consummate pro, Kelly shrugs off the miss, snaps her gum and walks out of the room without a backward glance.

The intern, proverbial low man on the medical totem pole, steps up next. His preparations to start the IV drag on for at least fifteen minutes. First he methodically lines up everything he needs for the task: the IV tubing, packs of alcohol wipes and stacks of 4 by 4 gauze pads. Next, he paces nervously, talking softly to himself. Is he praying? (*Good idea. Maybe I should join in*). Is he reciting the steps he memorized from a textbook? Suddenly I get a sinking feeling that since this is a teaching hospital, I might be his first tough stick. Ever.

With a flourish, the intern drapes my arm in blue cloth. Then he applies a topical cream to numb my left wrist; the kindness of his gesture warms my heart. Still, as I watch this twenty-something doctor-to-be, all that's missing is background music, something low and rhythmic with lots of percussion, building in slow beats to a crescendo. (Bumm-bumm-bumm-bumm-bumm-bumm-budda-bumm!).

I close my eyes, breathe deeply and tense for the worst. Despite all his good intentions and prep, the needle still hurts. But with an experienced nurse standing by to coach and cheerlead the entire process, (*hey, not bad for an intern*) an IV finally goes in. I hear congratulations all around. When I finally open my eyes, catch my breath and look around, I see crimson splotches staining the blue drape and red blood splatter on the floor near my feet. Blood. My blood and lots of it. Not unlike a crime scene. The good news is that antibiotics are flowing into me again, so maybe things are starting to look up.

Maybe not. Less than an hour later, as I sit in a chair reading a magazine in my room, still hooked up to the antibiotics, I idly scratch my head. Then feel the urge to scratch again. With each scratch, I feel small bumps rising under my fingers like mountains of mosquito bites. Hives! Angry, itchy hives popping up on my scalp, across my forehead, below my eyes, down my arms.

I buzz for the nurse. Scratch some more. When no one responds, I buzz again; the itchy feeling is getting intense. Uncomfortable. And still no response from anyone at the nurse's station. *This is insane*, I think to myself. How crazy is it that I'm having a reaction to the IV drugs and feel so helpless to do anything about it?

What are my choices? There's no way that I am going to pull out my brand new IV and I don't know the mechanics of stopping the drugs any other way. Minutes pass and by now I am raking both hands vigorously across my scalp to get some relief. Suddenly I feel dizzy, a little short of breath. Uh oh. I've read enough medical novels and watched enough doctor shows on TV to know that this is getting serious. I stand up, roll the IV stand out into the hall and yell as loud as I can: *Help! Nurse! Allergic reaction! Nurse! Help!*

Honestly, I was *this* close to screaming **STAT** too, but didn't. Blame it on episodes of *ER* and *Grey's Anatomy*. But in my own defense, when you are a cancer patient, shows like these are entertaining medical dramas with some helpful clinical info mixed in.

A dose of Benadryl takes care of the hives and they switch me to a new antibiotic. That works wonderfully well until my wrist starts swelling and they have to pull the IV. Next, a fourth year resident steps up to the plate and starts another line that crashes and burns the next day. The next strategy is to run a PICC line into a larger vein high on my left arm. Once installed, the PICC line pokes out from my arm like one of those pop up thermometers on a Perdue oven stuffer roaster. But the good news is that it's a line that could last for a couple of months. A PICC line sounds like a gift I should've been offered days ago, but I keep these bitter thoughts to myself.

My left arm is a mess; a rainbow-colored victim of intravenous complications, covered with green and blue and yellow colored bruises. In fact, my arm is in such bad condition that the day nurse begins applying hot compresses to bring down the swelling. She wets a compress, then wraps it in surgical tape before heating it in the kitchen microwave. The nurse brags to me that she was the one who came up with this great idea. Moments later, the steaming pack she places on my left arm is so scalding hot, it burns my wrist before I can knock it off. It lands on my thigh where it leaves an angry red mark along with a burned in pattern of lines from the surgical tape. There will be blisters by morning.

Anemia is the next complication. The daily bloodwork reveals that my red blood cell/hemoglobin count has plummeted, so they run the test again—the values are that low. Could the test be wrong? No, it's anemia. Why? "Trauma," says Dr. B. "Blood loss during surgery," he explains. "Of course your marrow was already compromised by eight rounds of chemotherapy."

On day six, I scribble the following desperate message in my journal addressed to no one in particular:

Help! I am trapped in an episode of ER and can't get out!

I think about taping this message to the door of my hospital room.

Time passes with agonizing slowness on the ward and I sense my hold on reality slowly slipping, day by day. (*Are you crazy if you think you might be crazy? Can you be aware of slowly losing your mind?*) I think strange thoughts. Like, suppose being a patient is my job. My mission. My destiny. My life's work, if you will. Could this be a legitimate form of full-time employment? You know, dress like the rest of the patients. Blend in. Observe and take notes. Make regular reports to the higher-ups. Get regular paychecks. A patient for hire. What a concept! Not unlike those professional passengers who fly around on airplanes and take notes on the quality of the in-flight beverage service on a short hop from Philly to Pittsburgh. I could do that, I think to myself. I could do that job very well.

As my mood swings from manic to depressed and back again, I write something in my journal that chills me when I stop and think about it: I feel like I am going to medical school the *really* hard way.

Before long, I start to learn staff names and shift schedules. (*Sarah comes on at 7. Eric has Tuesdays off*). The nurses allow me to come and go as I please; I'm a regular with open access to the supply closet where I pick up my own clean gowns, towels, sheets and blankets every morning. New patients come and go, check in, have surgery and go home, but not me; I never leave.

Gradually I even start to pick up details about other patients on the ward and try to chat with the nurses about them. "So how is the gall bladder in 662," I ask, making polite conversation, ignorant about violating confidentiality. "Did the hysterectomy go upstairs yet?" Before long I even help housekeeping strip and make up some beds on my hall; I am so anxious to be of some use to someone. To be acknowledged by anyone. One day an intern even catches me trying to log-on to the patient records computer outside my room and shoos me back to bed.

Yes, I am becoming a bad patient. A bored patient. An on-the-edge-of-crazy patient. Angry. Alienated. Alone and totally frustrated. Literally at my wit's end. I walk the halls compulsively three times a day on a rigid self-determined schedule, sometimes even wandering off the ward entirely as if planning a jailbreak. On day 7, out of desperation, my fruit basket gift and flower arrangements turn into arts and craft projects. I take them apart and create new still life designs on my window sills and counter tops. I experiment with colors and textures, fussing with the items to please my eye. (*Pears next to bananas. No, the apples go here*). Near the door to my room, I put out a bowl filled with gummy bear candy hoping to lure people in to visit with me.

In one extremely irrational moment, I look around my hospital room and decide that it would be lots roomier if I just took the leap, bit the financial bullet and put on an addition. I decide that I really need the space. I consider whether I could actually recoup my investment at time of sale.

In less than one week's time, how is it possible that my life has become so small and self-contained, shrunken down to the size of one small hospital room (w/bath, dropped ceiling, sixth floor view)?

"When can I go home?" I beg Dr. B. on the eve of day 8.

"Not for another couple of days," says Dr. B. When my eyes fill with tears, the plastic surgeon finally loses patience with me.

"We need to fight the infection," he says sternly. "This is very serious. I don't want to have to take you back into the operating room to work on the flap again. If this infection doesn't clear up, I just may have to. Then he says the words that finally make some sense to me. "We are not trying to punish you."

When Dr. B. leaves the room, I play back his words in my head a few times to make some sense of them. Like a good surgeon, Dr. B has cut right to the heart of the matter. Punishment. But here's the thing: if they are not punishing me, then what exactly are they doing? He should try to see things through my eyes. It all feels like punishment. One bad thing after another. By now, I have had more than enough.

Yes, I feel like a prisoner of war and their plan to torture me is working: dress me in a rag that snaps and ties in the back. Knock me out, cut me open, stitch me up. Keep me on my back for 48 hours without moving. Feed me horrible food. Disturb my sleep three times a night to check my vitals. Separate me from work, from home, from friends and family, from everything near and dear to me. Poke me with needles over and over and over again. Make me bleed. Profusely. Screw up my antibiotics. For good measure, give me second degree burns. And then, for the ultimate insult, don't let me shower or wash my hair for a week. That should do the trick.

By the morning of Day 8, at 6:45 am, when Dr. B's medical residents arrive for their regularly scheduled morning rounds, they peek in my room and see me curled up on the bed in a fetal position, pale, listless, feverish and unresponsive. It took eight days to whip the fight out of me, but it's clear that the process has worked. I have given up.

The team immediately goes into a huddle to discuss the dramatic change in the patient's condition. I overhear them repeating the phrase, "cabin fever."

By noon, I am discharged and on my way home.

THAT LUCKY GUY

Some intern christened me *post-op-who-walks-*
with-three-drains, but in twenty-five steps I'm
past the nursing station, ice machine and
laundry room; ten steps more and I'm home free-
off the ward, shuffling by on-call cells with
MDs-to-be asleep in their bunkbeds.
Breathless, I reach my goal—the P.T. ramp
surrounded by floor-to-ceiling windows
sealed against smells of spring. Yes, seasons changed
during my eight day incarceration.
Outside, six stories down, magnolia trees
dressed in pink-white wings guard a vagrant snug
in coarse newspaper blankets; my envy
seethes: *that lucky guy, he found a way out.*

Every Ride
in the Park

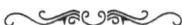

The words are purposes.
The words are maps.
I came to see the damage that was done
and the treasures that prevail.
—Adrienne Rich, "Diving Into the Wreck"

Everyone who is born holds dual citizenship, in the
kingdom of the well and in the kingdom of the sick.
Although we all prefer to use only the good passport,
sooner or later each of us is obliged, at least for a
spell, to identify ourselves as citizens of that other place.
—Susan Sontag, *Illness as Metaphor*

Breast Cancer Support Meeting Tonight & Refreshments Will Be Served

The drug rep pulls goodies
from a large shopping bag.
Struggles with a dull knife.
Cuts lengths of string
wrapped around
two white bakery boxes.

With a flourish, he lifts the lids,
opens twin treasure chests of sweets.
Reveals a fruit covered torte
draped in pineapple circles,
blood red strawberries and sliced bananas,
a cream filled cake
shiny with icing glaze.
And for the calorie counters,
a platter of ripe melon balls
ready to dive into lemon yogurt dip.

He works his buffet,
artfully arranges napkins, plates and forks-
a self-conscious host
fussing, folding, fidgeting,
anxious for his guests to arrive.

The first woman walks into the meeting room.
The drug rep jumps to attention.
Asks the obvious:

Are you a breast cancer survivor?

Before she can answer
floodgates open,
his questions spill out,
a torrent of medicalese:
Lumpectomy?
Mastectomy?
Bilateral?
Reconstruction?
Lymph nodes?
Metastatic?
Adjuvant treatment?
Chemo?
AC?
CMF?
CAF?
Tamoxifen?
Arimidex?

She listens open-mouthed and mute.
Her brain spins with unspoken questions:
Is this how we sing Getting-to-Know-You in Cancerland?
Should I begin my organ recital right on cue?
Shall I unbutton my shirt?
Does he need a quick peek?
Are breast cancer battle scars my ticket to eat?

He stops.
So does her angry mind chatter.
They face each other
Count off a silent beat.
She needs to answer him
Nothing more than this:

I've been on every ride in the park

The ice in her voice,
her down turned mouth,
halt a conversation
that never had a chance to start.

DELETERIOUS MUTATION

Deleterious. Such a musical five syllable word. I love the sound of language, and truly these eleven letters form a word that I could almost sing in the shower.

I tentatively say it out loud: *deleterious.* A lilting series of sounds rolling off the tongue—a word, quite honestly, that at first doesn't sound that scary at all. But the dictionary definition suggests otherwise: *injurious to health, harmful, derived from the Greek—a word meaning 'destroyer.'*

I am sitting in the doctor's office in a chair facing her desk. *Here's your copy of the test results,* she says. I look at what she has handed me and see the word *deleterious* sitting right next to the very threatening noun *mutation* and together those two words shout at me in a loud, ugly way. They are just two words, but together they form a nasty phrase that accurately describes me, who I am, who I've suddenly become, my new CancerLand identity.

Deleterious mutation. These are the words printed on a navy blue pocketed folder labeled *Understanding Your Genetic Test Result* that my doctor has just handed me. I can't help but notice that the BRAC Analysis folder is illustrated with a photograph in the upper left corner of an extremely sane looking, quite attractive middle-aged woman; she wears a pale purple sweater set that brings out the blue of her perfectly made-up eyes. She may be my new best friend at some point in the near future, a potential role model perhaps, the person I might hope to one day see looking back at me in the mirror now that I know what I know. But she is definitely *not* me, not now.

At this moment in time, we have absolutely nothing in common, not a single thing to talk about.

I think back to my last appointment with this doctor. How we chatted briefly after the physical exam. I was casually handing over my co-pay at the front desk when she suggested that I get genetic testing done. I wasn't the least bit interested. *I'm almost ten years out from diagnosis*, I argued. *I have no children. There's no family history.* Still the doctor insisted that it was in my best interests to get the test done. *The results will impact how all your doctors follow you*, she said. Then she told me that the lab tech was great with 'tough sticks' like me and had time right now to take my blood. I reluctantly agreed and moments later surrendered my left arm.

That was three weeks ago and now the results are in. I have tested positive for the BRCA2 mutation. On the paper clearly marked patient copy, under the interpretation column, there's that word again, this time in heavy bold print: **deleterious.**

The doctor looks through my file as she starts discussing possible next steps. *Remind me . . . which breast did you lose?* she asks, as if I have inadvertently misplaced a set of car keys and for some reason can't get my hands on them. *Right breast*, I reply. *Remind me*, she repeats . . . *you're the one who had the TRAM, right?*

No. I'm the lat flap, I say, wondering how much effort it would have taken for the doctor to review my file before this meeting began. Then I wonder, who is the other patient that she has confused me with? I find myself thinking about this other woman, this other breast cancer survivor, this unidentified woman who had a TRAM flap reconstruction, who probably wouldn't appreciate being confused with me either. I wonder if this other patient ever becomes impatient with the doctor, or on the verge of anger—feeling the way I'm feeling right now. *This is becoming quite a deleterious genetic counseling session*, I think to myself, *one that is starting to aggravate me.*

The empathy that I had felt in all of my previous dealings with this doctor seems totally absent today. And that's a damn shame because some TLC would've made this particular CancerLand chapter a lot easier to handle. I feel like I've just been diagnosed with cancer all over again.

One option is to have a second mastectomy, she says and starts quoting the statistics. I see the doctor's lips moving as she forms the words and can't help but mentally hit a mute button to silence her. *No, that's not an option*, I interrupt. *I don't think the ultimate benefit outweighs the risks associated with another surgery, not to mention the emotional trauma of a second mutilating procedure. Plus, don't we have lots of ways to maintain close surveillance on my remaining breast?* I fight the urge to cover my left side with both hands; how can I possibly explain how incredibly protective I am of my remaining breast? Am I a fool to expect that a woman doctor might totally "get" that?

That's true, she says, *I understand*, she says, but honestly I don't think she really understands at all. The two breasts she was born with are still where they are supposed to be, on her chest, front and center, projecting symmetrically with an attractive bit of cleavage showing at the spot where her silk blouse is stylishly undone an extra button.

Well then, she continues, all business, *you should think about having your ovaries removed to minimize the risk of ovarian cancer.* The doctor quotes another bunch of statistics just then and I feel my body start to go numb in places. There must be a shocked expression on my face because suddenly the doctor tries a more personal touch. *You know*, she says, *I met with a group of my girlfriends last month and we were talking about breast cancer. The statistics say 'one in eight' women will get the disease. We looked around, counted heads and realized that it could be one of us. Would you believe that I just heard that one of my friends from that group of ladies was just diagnosed? Stage two breast cancer with lymph node involvement*, she says.

Why is she telling me this story? I am puzzled. I sense the doctor's palpable relief that she in fact was *not* the one-in-eight in her circle of girlfriends. So I have to wonder, has this doctor has ever had a sick day in her life? Or experienced anything more traumatic than a broken nail or a flat tire? I can't control these ugly thoughts that keep popping up and bumping into one another in my head as I look at my doctor. But I exert enough self-control to not say a word out loud; I truly don't know how to respond. What great insight or meaningful life lesson can I come up with after hearing about her friend? And then in a flash, it all becomes crystal clear what her anecdote says to me in the most personal way possible: I am in fact the loser in the genetic sweepstakes. No question. *The Big Loser.* I am the one-in-eight.

The genetic testing results are in fact a gift that has finally answered the big question, 'how did I get breast cancer?' That has been an unresolved issue since my diagnosis. Now I know what I know: it wasn't a neighborhood golf course on Long Island sprayed with DDT in the fifties that was to blame. It was a gene (*bad, bad, deleteriously mutated gene*) that turned on and started a tumor growing. I can be as angry as I want to be and it still won't change a thing. The genetic testing yields significant data and it would serve me to accept the news. I will sign up for lots of office visits every year with at least three different doctors and put up with endless numbers of tests rather than hop up on the table for more surgery; that's my choice and it feels right for me right now. Given the choice, I'll take calm acceptance over righteous anger any day of the week . . .

As these thoughts spin through my head, suddenly I also realize that I am this doctor's last patient on a Friday afternoon in the summertime and our counseling session is over. *I will call your breast surgeon. But not today. Most folks are already headed down the shore for the weekend,* the doctor says. And that message travels across her desk to me loud and clear. No additional translation is necessary. If I would just get up and leave, she would be moving in the very same direction.

THIS IS A TEST

In school, you're taught a lesson and then given a test.
In life, you're given a test that teaches you a lesson.
—Tom Bodett

I am lying flat on my back in a dimly lit room, naked and draped from the waist down. My knees are spread apart. There are two fat pillows wedged under my butt to tilt my pelvis upwards. A technician passes me a probe between my legs, and using clinically correct terminology, tells me in no uncertain terms where to stick it. Then she deftly maneuvers the probe around inside of me in a pattern that immediately brings to mind the stick shift of an old red Volkswagen Rabbit that I used to drive way back when. This is humiliating. This is dehumanizing. This hurts. This is a test.

I hate this.

Did I actually say that out loud? Or just think it to myself? I don't know for sure. And looking over at the tech doesn't give me any clue. Out of the corner of my eye, I watch her focus intently on her computer screen, feel her downshift from third to second gear (*ouch!*) and then hear the mouse double-click.

The scene is so familiar; I have been on this table twice before. And one thing is certain—this is one of those tests that I dread from start to finish. No doubt about it. I hate this surreal-sticky-skin-crawling-nasty-trans-vaginal ultrasound test that I have to take twice a year. Why don't they upgrade it to include a hot shower along with a glass of chilled white wine on the way out the door?

Couldn't hurt. Might help.

Tests. Way back when, B.C. (before cancer), tests were so simple, weren't they? A predictable process that went something like this: a teacher taught the class for a time and then announced the upcoming date of the test. Next, the teacher shared important details with the students. What topics the test would cover. What form the test would be: essay, short answer, true/false. You studied, (admit it: some of us more than others), managed your test anxiety, took the test and waited to get your grade. End of story. Of course, in college, there was the added drama of larger classes, harder tests and those foolish little blue books to scribble your essays into. But somehow we all learned to play the take-the-test game and the earth continued to spin on its axis.

Tests. B.C., that was all the word meant to me—paper, pencil, getting good grades. But now, living day-to-day, year after year in CancerLand, with the real anxiety of managing a BRCA-2 deleterious mutation, when it comes to tests, (new tests, more tests, with or without contrast), I am struggling with a new reality. Instead of agreeing to more surgery, I've got my Doctor's notes, insurance I.D. card and co-payments in hand. I'm now a somewhat reluctant frequent flyer for tests. Truth be told, I am whining more and tolerating much less when it comes to tests these days. So while my G.P.A. isn't suffering as a result, my patience, along with my sense of humor, are both being seriously challenged.

A week later, I am lying face down on my stomach on a platform with cutouts to cradle my various body parts. *This is my first Breast MRI,* I confess to the technician. *Please be gentle with me.* My initial impression is this: breasts are round in shape, but for a Breast MRI, your boobs are supposed to drop neatly into two side-by-side rectangles. Go figure.

My face is nested in what looks and feels like a catcher's mitt. There's a hole in the middle to help me breathe through my nose or mouth.

(*Just like when you get a massage*, says the technician). Bright orange earplugs pop into place, followed by a headset on top. (*You need these or else it will be too loud in there*, says the technician). Then she takes my arms and stretches them uncomfortably over my head so that my fingers touch. Finally, she places a rubber ball in my right hand. (*This is your stress ball*, says the technician. *Try not to move, okay?*).

Stress ball? (*Should I squeeze it when I feel anxious? Or is it a panic button for when I freak out? Will you stop the MRI if I signal you? Will you let me out? Then will I have to go back inside to finish the test?*) I don't get the chance to ask any of these questions because the platform starts moving slowly backwards, delivering me, face down, feet first inside the MRI tube. In a panic, I quickly close my eyes and decide in that moment to handle the stress ball delicately, like a fragile egg that might break under the slightest pressure.

That will be my last somewhat rational thought for the next twenty-five minutes.

The clicking noises begin and through the racket I hear a male voice calling my name. Everything is so muffled by the earplugs and the headset and the pounding of my heart, it sounds like a man hollering under water. (*Who is that? Why is someone trying to talk to me now? Why didn't they say what they had to say before I went inside the MRI?*) I finally reply and acknowledge the second technician and he thankfully stops yelling at me.

The test launches to a land far, far away—a land of loud noise. Large waves of sound build up and wash over me, rumble around, inside and through me, again and again. Clicking sounds change to clanging sounds change to Star Wars lightsabers slashing. Every so often, the male tech's voice intrudes (*Six minutes this time*). Then the cycle of noise begins again. Clicking. Clanging. Beneath the noise, there's a voice in my head screaming, *I don't want to be here. I want this to be over and done with already.* I try to breathe slowly in and out, in and out. I try to separate from my body and disappear to some happy place far away from here. I try to fight the panic of feeling buried alive. I try not to squeeze the stress ball. I try I try. I try. I try. I try. I try. I try. I try. I try. I try. I try. I try. I try. I try. I try. I try. I-

Suddenly there's silence—a blessed absence of noise. The table slowly moves me headfirst into the light. I gratefully open my eyes. The MRI technician is at my side, eager to get me up and out of the machine and into the dressing room. But I feel dizzy and altered, disoriented and weak in the knees. *Give me a moment, will you please?* I ask the technician, as I slowly sit up and swing my legs over the edge of the table. *I have to ask you a question,* I say. *When you did your training to become an MRI tech, did they make you take this test?*

No way, she says. *In my class, we were all way too claustrophobic to handle a Breast MRI.*

They say laughing is good for your health. According to Norman Cousins, it just might cure what ails you. Laughing feeds your soul and lifts your spirits. After two Fridays in a row visiting my local imaging center, taking my scheduled spring tests, this was as funny as it got. In fact, after the MRI, once my head cleared, I giggled all the way home. Bottom line—here's what I know for sure: a good cleansing laugh and a righteous rant about tests I *have* to but don't *want* to take, will probably keep me going until it's time for me to jump back up on the table to be tested again.

And that may be the very best that I can do.

LOWEST POINT

After one of my many cancer surgeries, I woke up hungry.

Ravenously hungry.

Give-me-something-to-eat-now-or-else hungry. The way my stomach was growling, you would think that I had been fasting for weeks, not just since midnight the night before being admitted to the hospital.

But now it was after 5 pm, I was out of recovery and back in my room. By my count, that meant two whole meals missed. Clearly, I felt compelled to make up for lost time. That explains why, when a nurse walked by my room nibbling on a bag of vending machine cookies, I wasn't shy about asking for what I needed.

Your dinner tray has been ordered, she said. *You really should wait for it to arrive.*

Well, that answer just wasn't good enough for me. Plus the hospital food wasn't nearly as tempting as chocolate chip cookies. (As post-op patients go, I know I can be very pushy and on occasion, incredibly persuasive).

Maybe you can guess what happened next.

Two chocolate chip cookies later, I got sick. So sick in fact that I hurled with gusto across the full length of my hospital bed. This was puking as an Olympic event, with points given for quantity and distance. The sheets, blankets and my hospital gown were completely covered with vomit.

Oh my God, look at me. I'm pathetic, I sobbed, all the while trying in vain to help the nurse clean up the soiled bedding. *Pathetic! Please forgive me. I'm so sorry. Things can't get much worse than this . . .*

In CancerLand, when you hit your lowest point, clearly the only direction left to go is up.

And sometimes at that terrible moment, when you hit rock bottom, the Universe sends a signal that lights your path, and offers you a faint glimmer of hope.

Other times, not so much.

You just might find yourself slogging through a proverbial sea of clichés trying to get to that better place because this is what you'll hear everyone saying:

- it's always darkest before the dawn
- things will turn around
- this is just a bump in the road; nothing more than a temporary setback
- hang in there—you will get through this

Winston Churchill had an interesting way of looking at low points in life. But let the record show that he probably wasn't thinking about CancerLand when he said, "if you're going through hell, keep going."

In my case, the sympathetic nurse who cleaned me up that night, comforted me with a cliché of her own that I've never forgotten:

Years from now, you will look back on this and laugh, she said.

And what do you know? She was right. I do. Still.

CALL YOUR NURSE

Call . . . your . . . nurse.

The mechanical voice coming out of the rapid infuser wakes me from a drugged sleep with a start.

Where the hell am I? I'm not sure. And the room doesn't offer many clues. None that I can make sense of anyway. There's blackness around me except for a small bit of light seeping in from under the closed door. Peering around the room, my eyes gradually adjust to the dark. At first, nothing looks even vaguely familiar and I feel disturbed and alone and panicky. But after a tense minute and a few deep breaths, I begin to get my bearings and try to talk myself down from the ledge.

(*Hospital. Okay. The hospital. Surgery this morning. BRCA-2 Hysterectomy. That's right. I'm post-op. Great. Great. That's just great. I'm in the hospital. And the surgery's done*).

It feels late. Maybe it's the middle of the night. But I can't be sure since I don't see a clock on the wall and my sense of time is totally twisted. I swallow. I'm so dry, so incredibly thirsty, so empty and hungry; my throat feels sore and raggedy.

There's a remote control with a button near my right hand. Morphine for pain. I remember that now. The nurse explained that to me before I went down for surgery. I push the button three times.

By the time I count to ten the panic's gone. No more pain. I feel my edges soften. I'm still post-op. I'm still alone in the dark in a strange place. But what's different now is that I just don't *care* as much.

Feeling much more peaceful now, I tentatively grope under the covers and place my hands gently on the ON-Q pain pump the surgeon told me about. I move my hands sideways to find a small pillow resting on top of the thick surgical dressing that covers my abdomen from hip to hip. While I continue my post-op investigation, compression stockings wrapped around each of my calves mechanically fill up with air and deflate, fill up and deflate, over and over and over and over and over . . .

That's when I hear the voice again.

Call . . . your . . . nurse.

Maybe this is something new, I think to myself, looking over at the rapid infuser parked on the left side of my hospital bed. Even in the dark, I can see the outlines of two bags of intravenous drugs hanging from the pole and follow the IV lines trailing downwards to a spot on my left arm. I haven't spent this much time up close and personal with a rapid infuser since my days in the Chemo Lounge, and I wonder if these gadgets have gone super high-tech now and can actually talk! Chances are one of the bags is empty and needs to be replaced. This all somehow makes perfect sense to me.

Then I hear that voice again, mechanical and insistent.

Call . . . your . . . nurse.

I want to be a good post-op patient. In fact, I want to be the best post-op patient ever, so the search for the nurse call button begins. It must be near the bed somewhere, right within reach, *right under my nose probably, big as life,* I think to myself, *so let's see if I can find it.* After all, the machine is telling me that I've got to call my nurse!

Holding my pillow across my incision with my right hand, I feel around the edges of the bed in the dark to hunt for a remote control attached to a thick cord. I feel a cord off to my right and reach in that direction. *Ouch!* The incision pulls painfully up the middle and at the same time the IV line reins me in from my left side. The compression stockings throw my body off balance from the knees down. After a few minutes of awkward exertion, I am halfway off the bed, unable to move in either direction.

Stuck. Horribly stuck. Like a turtle on its back.

And that's the way a nurse finds me when the shift changes a short time later. She immediately calls in another nurse, they grab the sheets on either side and one-two-three efficiently pull me back to the center of the bed. *Where were you trying to go?* the nurses ask me. *What were you trying to do?*

I am ready with my explanation

The rapid infuser kept talking to me. It said I was supposed to call a nurse so I . . .

I stop talking when I see one of the nurses biting down on her lip to keep from laughing. She quickly turns and leaves the room. The sound of her giggling echoes down the hallway as she heads to the nurse's station.

Don't feel too badly, the other nurse says, trying to comfort me. *It's just all those drugs in your system.*

My chart states that I was released on post-op day three with a prescription for Percoset ('take 1 tablet by mouth every 4 hours if needed for pain.') The surgeon had given me the prescription during pre-op testing and I had gone over to the neighborhood Rite Aid a week before surgery to get it filled. I had carefully placed the bottle of pills on the bottom shelf of my medicine cabinet where it would be easy to reach once I came home from the hospital. But you know what? After my close encounter with a talking rapid infuser, I learned my lesson well.

I never broke the seal on the bottle.

CancerLand in the First Person

I am diagnosed
I'm numb
I cry
I curse
I blame
I pray
I bargain
I float
I fight
I hide

I am cut
I'm sliced
I'm stitched
I bleed
I leak
I'm drained
I reach
I peek
I grieve
I heal

I am poisoned
I'm nauseous
I'm slow
I'm stupid
I shed
I'm bald
I'm wigged

I walk
I disappear
I heal

I am radiated
I'm placed
I'm marked
I'm blasted
I'm burned
I bitch
I redden
I itch
I peel
I heal

I am reconstructed
I'm filled
I'm stretched
I'm filled
I'm stretched
I'm filled
I'm stretched
I peek
I pass
I heal

I am recovering
I write
I read
I coach
I plant
I grow
I breathe
I live
I'm feeling
I'm healing

Plastic Surgeon Photo Shoot

I double click to open my journal—a computer folder on my desktop filled with lots and lots of Word files, some dating back to the day my CancerLand journey began. These are files packed full of details of everything that has happened to me—day by day, one doctor's appointment after another—since I was diagnosed with breast cancer.

And as I glance at some text on the screen, one journal entry catches my eye, holds my attention and refuses to let go. Ten long years later, one particularly painful visit to a plastic surgeon still resonates in memory . . .

Good, that's very good, the plastic surgeon says, his face totally hidden behind the camera. *What's good?* she thinks to herself. *How I look?* There's a brief delay as the doctor focuses, another as the electronic flash unit whirrs and recycles.

Pictures. Plastic surgeons need to take pictures. Lots of pictures. Before pictures. Post-reconstruction pictures. Expect-multiple-revisions-because-cosmesis-is-a-lengthy-process pictures.

So she faces the camera, flushed and red-faced, for a seemingly endless number of medical photographs. She poses as the doctor directs her to: naked to the waist, standing in front of a seamless black velvet background. While she feels exposed and vulnerable, truly uncomfortable in her own skin, she doesn't say a word. But the unspoken dialogue in her head is another matter entirely.

Let's finish this already. You're not a photographer shooting a Vogue cover, for crying out loud, and I'm sure as hell no supermodel, she thinks to herself.

Then she shivers, suddenly imagining what these photographs of her upper body will look like. Cringes knowing that there will now be a permanent record somewhere of her extreme disfigurement: a purplish biopsy scar . . . the pale pink round bump of the port on her left side . . . patches of radiated skin burned to various shades of pale pink and light brown.

Truth be told, lately she has purposely avoided looking too closely at her naked body in the full-length mirror on the back of the bathroom door when she steps out of the shower every morning. There might be lots of good reasons why.

Over the past 18 months of medical procedures, radiation treatments, repeated breast surgeries and failed attempts at reconstruction, there have been so many physical changes. (the winding path of her mastectomy scar . . . the softball shaped right breast mound that sits grotesquely high on her chest, nudging her collarbone). Disturbing and dramatic changes to a body she lives in, but these days doesn't recognize as her own.

She hasn't mastered the breast cancer survivor's fine art of looking in the mirror—each and every time the bandages are removed, following yet another surgical procedure—without crying tears of disappointment and frustration.

Then she hears the camera shutter click again. She blinks at the bright light of the flash. *I am shooting you from the neck down,* the plastic surgeon says.

Well, that's good to know, she thinks to herself, *because I am definitely not smiling for the camera.*

89

In fact, at this point, her mind chatter is so loud that she almost doesn't hear the doctor's mumbled comments as he scrutinizes his "tough case" of the day through the camera's viewfinder. *Anything we do for you*, the plastic surgeon says, *anything will be an improvement.*

RECONSTRUCTION

She stands on a low stool
wearing blue surgical booties
and a dazed expression,
limp cotton gown at her feet.
Plastics men with purple magic markers
(permanent pointy tip)
circle her, chatter in matching mint green scrubs,
slowly map the scalpel's winding path
with purple spots and sketchy lines.
They connect dots, front and back,
mark pale skin sorely branded,
burned and scarred.
She senses their plot and plan
from a distant place.
Her hands first flutter nervously at her sides
then clutch and clench,
open closed, open closed
pushing shame and anger
in hot surges, up to stain her cheeks red.
Naked and fierce, no pockets hide her fists.
She poses on her pedestal,
spins around slow,
no twinge of fear, no prayer of hope,
mute—a block of damaged marble
impatient for an artist's sharp blade
to set her spirit free.

REVISION

I am in touch with the fantasy, the technicolor fantasy spinning through my head as I walk into the doctor's office on a Thursday afternoon, twenty minutes before my scheduled appointment. It's my very own summer-blockbuster-technicolor-plastic surgery-reconstruction-revision fantasy, and it goes like this:

I see myself sitting on the edge of the examining table covered with that crinkly white paper that makes crackly noises as I fidget from side to side, wearing a salmon colored gown that I hold closed with two sweaty hands.

The surgeon knocks twice, and walks in the room head down, intently reviewing my medical file. She looks up. Our eyes lock for a moment. The doctor has a cool professional smile on her face, gentle and reassuring. She assesses me with a quick head to toe glance, matching the words in the patient file with the nervous person sitting in front of her.

Finally she asks in a kind voice, *What brings you here today?* That's my cue to open the gown with a dramatic flourish, exposing my reconstructed right side.

It looks bad. It feels bad, I will no doubt say, averting my eyes, blood rushing to my cheeks. *Like a lightbulb screwed into my chest. It took two years and six surgeries done by three different doctors to make me to look this way.* I will dutifully recite doctors' names and hospital affiliations, surgery dates, procedures and problems from memory, using the most clinically accurate terms I know. (lumpectomy, dirty margins, mastectomy, failed expansion with saline implant, latissimus dorsi flap with saline implant, multiple post-operative complications).

At this point, I will probably think about lightening up the mood in the room a bit, with a joke or snappy comment; (*Hey, doc, I guess you've figured it out by now that I went to medical school the really hard way, huh?*). This is actually one of my favorite lines to use with new doctors during an initial visit, but maybe I need to hold back this time. After so many years, it might be high time to let go of the CancerLand Comedian shtick already. (*How's that working for you?*)

Instead I will probably pause, take a deep breath, and gear up to ask the big question—a question so huge that I have to save it for the big finish: *Can you make it any better?*

There. I will have said it. Put it out in the open. Asked simply and directly for what I need. No begging. No whining. No pleading words like, *Can you help me? Can you? Would you? Now? Please?*

The technical term for what I'm interested in getting from my new plastic surgeon is a "revision," which is in fact the strangest word imaginable to describe my heart's desire since my mastectomy—as if my chest were a tenth grade student's five paragraph essay that is in screaming need of a major rewrite. (*details lacking, sparse in parts, unbalanced but a noble effort nonetheless! Keep trying! I can't wait to see the next one!*) The gold standard in the world of breast reconstruction is symmetry, but when it comes to reconstructing radiated skin, all bets are off.

Despite the odds, even after all these years, I'm strangely hopeful. Maybe number seven will be the charm. Maybe my lucky number seven reconstruction revision procedure will do the trick. What a crap shoot! The truth is there are moments when I weaken and can't quite believe that I am ready to hop back up on the operating table again for another surgery.

So here's the rest of the fantasy. The sorts of things I imagine telling a female plastic surgeon, believing that, since she was born with the same basic equipment, she just might understand where I'm coming from . . .

I dream about wearing a tank top without worrying about the neckline slipping down to reveal the 'pot hole' where the radiation left a sizeable dent. I dream of wearing a real bra, a plain old bra (Victoria's Secret be damned), with two cups that I fill out equally, just like millions of other women every day, all over the world, dressing on autopilot, while they think about other, far more important things they need to get done.

I dream of trying on clothes in Loehmann's, right out in the open, in the big dressing room, without feeling self-conscious. I dream that I stare at my reflection in the full-length mirror and smile with satisfaction because the clothes actually fit, both sides match and they are on sale to boot!

But most of all I dream of taking a shower and looking down, feeling comfortable with my middle aged body—feeling whole and attractive again.

Hey, it's my reconstruction revision fantasy and I'm sticking with it! I will carry it gift wrapped, tied up nice with a big pink bow (naturally) to my new plastic surgeon's office and wait patiently for her response to my question, "can you make it any better?"

Can she? Will she? How much longer do I need to wait?

In fact, my actual visit to the plastic surgeon played out much like my fantasy, and I'm thrilled to report that I will in fact be going under the knife again for a revision to my reconstruction.

Wish me luck! It's just one more step in my CancerLand journey . . .

ME AND MY VAMPIRE

I grip the envelope tightly in my hand. The words *Pre-admission Testing* are block printed in black ink across the front. Inside there's a form already filled out with my name, birthday and date of surgery, along with a long list of mysterious acronyms and medical abbreviations.

Time for a little pep talk. I can't help but think about what's ahead for me—another major surgery with weeks of recovery. But this morning, what's happening today will be a piece of cake by comparison. Easy as can be. No big deal. After all, I should be a total pro by now after years of practice, right? Anyone like me who has spent so much time in CancerLand knows the pre-op drill by heart and it goes like this: get your pre-admission testing done, or else no surgery for you.

But this hospital is new to me; I don't know my way around and that always makes me a little jumpy. I hate getting lost. So I mentally review my instructions: *show the ladies at the information desk this envelope*, the surgeon's office manager said. *They will tell you where you need to go in the hospital to get your pre-op testing done.*

Sounds simple enough. But preparing emotionally for another big surgery is much more challenging. Being here today is certainly the next step in facing up to the reality of surgery #8 next week.

I grip the envelope tightly in my hand as I walk across the parking lot, enter the hospital lobby and locate the information desk. A grey-haired volunteer smiles in my direction. *Pre-admission testing?* I ask.

Make a right, go down the hall make a left turn after the elevators and look for the sign, says the woman with a hospital ID pinned to her blouse.

I grip the envelope and stroll past the gift shop and up to the first sign on the wall—a Kafkaesque affair that has at least fifteen different locations listed, with arrows pointing this way and that. Finally, at the end of a long hallway, I locate the Pre-admission Testing office and walk in. I try to catch the eye of the woman sitting at her desk intently tapping on her keyboard and studying her computer screen. She barely acknowledges me as she reaches for my paperwork.

After a quick scan of the form, she shakes her head. *No, you aren't registered yet*, the woman says with finality, before robotically reciting directions back to the main lobby of the hospital.

Within minutes I am back to square one, standing at the information desk, with impatient thoughts running through my head (*you can't get there from here*) asking for directions to the admissions office to register (*information I should have been told **yesterday***). Before long, I have multiple copies of the pre-admission testing form in hand and walk back to the pre-admission testing office to try again.

I try a little humor, no doubt to ease my own anxiety. *Hey, remember me? It's like déjà vu, all over again*, I say.

The pre-admission testing lady is a tough audience, no doubt about it. Without cracking a smile, she takes my paperwork, time-stamps it and points to a door. *EKG and bloodwork there,* she says.

Feel the love.

I walk into the waiting room. There's a machine on the wall that spits out slips of paper, (*now serving number 86*) just like in a bakery. I reach out ready to press down the red lever, when I read a nearby sign that proclaims, **Pre-admission Testing Patients Do Not Need to Take a Number!!!**

The three exclamation marks on the sign do their work well. No number for me. I slouch down in a molded plastic chair and silently think to myself, *how is it possible after ten years in CancerLand that I still feel like such a stranger in a strange land?*

I hear my name badly mispronounced over the loudspeaker. No one else responds, so I get up and walk into an examination room and stretch out on the table. After some sticker placement and untangling of wires, the technician finishes the EKG. In seconds it seems. Certainly in less time than it took me to walk back and forth to the Information Desk.

Getting tubes of blood out of me will be more of a challenge. But, then again, it always is. *Sorry, I know that I'm a tough stick*, I say to the technician. One butterfly, one painful stick, one swollen arm, and the tech graciously admits defeat.

Come with me, she says with a smile. *I'm taking you to see The Vampire.*

I follow the technician into a back room where a dark-haired man dressed in blue scrubs is standing up, peering at a computer screen on the counter.

I've got a tough stick for you, says the technician to The Vampire.

I sit in the chair and offer up my bare left arm to The Vampire. He looks down and studies my arm intently. While he concentrates on my veins, I check him out: (*Good news; no fangs*) luminous brown eyes with dark super long eyelashes, an ornamental red mark on his forehead between his eyebrows. I look at his exotically handsome face and decide that he could be the lead actor in a Bollywood feature if he wasn't already the star of the pre-admissions testing department.

Why do they call you The Vampire? I ask.

Because I like tough sticks, he says slowly in a heavy foreign accent.

What's your secret to hitting the tough sticks? I ask.

No secret really. I'm just the best. Trust me, it is a very spiritual thing, he says stroking the skin near the crook of my arm.

I make a fist out of habit. *There's no need*, says The Vampire. *Open your hand. Relax. Close your eyes and breathe and I will get the three tubes of blood we need, one-two-three-no problem. Trust me. Trust me . . .*

His soft voice lulls me and sends me to a calmer place.

He glances down at my paperwork, *Oh, I see that your birthday is coming up later this month.*

He begins to sing softly and even with my eyes closed, I join him: *Happy Birthday to you, Happy Birthday to you, Happy Birthday, Alysa Cummings, Happy Birthday to you.*

I am done, he says, holding up the three vials of blood, *and this is your birthday present.*

I open my eyes and can't help but smile. Birthday present? I'll say it is! A gift of no pain. No bruises. My pre-admission testing completed. Thank you doesn't begin to cover it.

Minutes later, I am halfway across the hospital parking lot on my way to the car before I realize that I forgot to ask The Vampire an essential question.

I couldn't help but wonder—were *his* eyes closed too?

Impatient Patient

(for Julia Darling, in appreciation)

Such an impatient patient . . .
I'm waiting for
gas to pass,
stitches to dissolve,
and visiting nurses
to knock
on my front door.

One week post-op
I'm waiting for
path reports
(*good news, please*),
permission to drive
and stacks of get well cards
in my mailbox.

Slow torture
mending day by day,
(heal me, free me),
weary me—waiting for
my "new normal"
to appear
(whatever the hell that means . . .).

The surgeon counsels patience;
Take six weeks or so:
recuperate.

(*sooner*, I beg, *faster*, I say).
impatient patient
I'm sick and tired
of recovery.

Give me
my strength,
my health,
my energy back!
impatient patient
I might just as well ask
seeds to grow,
buds to burst
and flowers to bloom
on my command.

A Country Far Away as Health

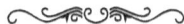

I have walked through many lives,
some of them my own,
And I am not who I was.
—Stanley Kunitz, "The Layers"

Dancing with NED*

I love NED.
He's a wonderful guest,
a great guy to live with,
a real nice fellow to have around.
NED's a busy man,
but I'll share him with my sisters.
May you and NED have
a long, happy life together!
Come on in and stay awhile, NED,
for as long as you want.
I need to meet NED.
I need NED in my life.
Enjoy your dance with NED
Tell him to save a
dance for me.
Let's visit Club NED soon.
Zippity-doo-dah, zippity-ay,
my oh my, NED has come here to stay;
N-E-D: I just love those three little letters.

*NED stands for "no evidence of disease; online cancer survivors
often refer to NED as a real person.

DONATIONS GRATEFULLY ACCEPTED

Donations. I'm a volunteer in charge of donations for a local office of a national cancer organization. So for a few hours every week, I sort through bags stuffed full of donations. Cancer-related types of donations to be exact: wigs, hats, scarves, bras and breast prostheses. Special items that cancer survivors often need and don't have the money (or insurance coverage) to buy. Things that help ladies look as good as they can after surgery and during cancer treatment.

Here's the drill: I empty a bag of donations onto a long table, hold up each item and evaluate: (*Would I wear this wig? Or is it too worn out to be recycled?*) Within minutes I have a pile of treasures that will eventually make their way into the hands (and in some cases onto the heads) of cancer patients who will make good use of them.

Donations. I've done this work for more than a year now and it has a way of making me smile. I like the feeling of serving fellow cancer survivors. It feels good to give back this way.

But on occasion as I have sifted through a bag of donations, my mind has wandered. (*Who wore this wig?*) And I have consciously tried to imagine the wig belonging to a woman like me, a cancer survivor happy to have finally finished chemo and radiation. A woman now well into recovery, deciding to donate her wig because her hair has grown back. I haven't wanted to think about other, sadder possibilities.

And that strategy has worked wonderfully well. Up until now, that is.

I spotted the bra first, poking out of the top of a brown Acme bag: pale pink, barely worn, folded in half, one cup neatly tucked inside the other. When I upended the bag, two wigs slid out: each short, brown, layered with auburn highlights. I continued to inventory the bag's contents: one silicone prosthesis (size 12), one lace trimmed sleeping cap, six headscarves (*one scarf caught my eye; silk paisley patterned and long enough to wrap around your head a few times. Wouldn't that look absolutely fierce with a pair of big silver hoop earrings?*). Finally, on the bottom of the bag, there was a donor note.

The cancer organization acknowledges all donations with a thank-you letter, so I opened the note and scanned it quickly for name and address information. That's when I read the message inside: *In memory of Susan P.*

I was stopped. Stopped cold. *Susan P. I know Susan P.* I instantly corrected myself. *I knew Susan P. before she died.* She was a member of my breast cancer support group.

Memories of Susan played back in my head—Susan telling stories about caring neighbors who checked in on her after surgery, Susan reading her first poem to the group with tears in her eyes, Susan on the phone from her hospital room trying to make sense of her recurrence—ending with the final image—a cold, rainy night at a local funeral home, waiting my turn to walk by her coffin and pay my respects to her family.

Donations. I'm a volunteer in charge of donations for a local office of a national cancer organization. So after I grabbed a tissue and wiped away the tears, I picked up a brush, shook out and styled the first wig and carefully anchored it on a mannequin head with a wig pin. Then I tied the silk paisley scarf around the mannequin's neck with a flourish. *For you, Susan*, I whispered. *For you, dear friend.*

THE LAST NOEL

for S.S.

Six years. I check the calendar and still can't quite believe my eyes.

Six years since *that* December—her last December.

Here's what I remember:

She and I were support group buddies who gradually turned into best friends. And like so many patients who find each other, forge a bond and travel through CancerLand together, we focused on getting through it as a team, one challenging day at a time: the doctor's appointments, the surgeries, the rounds of chemo, the seemingly endless wait for test results . . .

Until one day in late November when we heard the terrible news from her doctors. There was nothing left to do, they said; no new treatments to try. And her favorite time of year—Christmas—was right around the corner.

My friend told me she had a mission—to make it to Christmas. She told me in no uncertain terms that there was a big, long list of things that had to be done before December 25th. That's when I came up with a great idea. *Let me be your Hanukkah Elf,* I joked. *But since this is not my holiday, please be patient with me. Hey, I'm trainable and more than willing to do whatever I can to help.*

My friend was so organized that despite her fragile health, she had already finished her holiday shopping. Her spare bedroom was filled with all of the toys, sweaters, and assorted holiday tchotchkes that she planned to give to her family and friends. There was a proverbial mountain of gifts to be tagged and wrapped, all under my friend's watchful eye. Everything had to be "just so" for Christmas. Nothing less than perfect was acceptable. So with scissors in one hand and scotch tape in the other, I went to work. Hours later, the long dining room table was stacked end to end with presents wrapped in shiny red and green holiday paper.

Decorating the tree was the next challenge. *There's a first time for everything*, I said. *So where do I start?* I asked looking at the jumble of lights and boxes of sparkly ornaments on the floor in the den. My friend looked at me from her wheelchair parked on the other side of the room and shook her head in disbelief. *You really don't know how to decorate a Christmas tree?*

She silently pointed to a roll of wide ribbon on the coffee table. I picked it up and began to unwind it. **Noel, Noel, Noel**, I read aloud, admiring the shiny gold letters against the red background. *Anchor the ribbon near the top of the tree*, my friend said. *Now work the ribbon around the tree to your right, going in between the branches and keep going around and around and around . . .*

Look at me decorating a Christmas tree, I said to myself. *And not doing a bad job of it either.* Then I heard a sound behind me. Laughter. I turned around. My friend was laughing so hard that tears were running down her face. *What?* I asked. *Are you okay? What's so funny?*

Who. Is. Leon? My friend gasped between snorts of laughter. I looked up at the tree. The ribbon was wrapped around the tree, perfectly spaced between the branches, from top to bottom. Backwards. My friend continued to laugh. *Leon? Leon? Leon?*

When December rolls around on the calendar and I see Christmas trees on display, I can't help but remember my friend. She orchestrated an amazing, picture perfect, last Christmas and even taught a Hanukkah Elf the finer points of holiday tree decoration. What an amazing woman! What a wonderful friend! I still miss her and believe that I always will.

Six years later and memories from that day can still move me to tears, but somehow—and here's the thing, the best part—there's always a smile on my face at the very same time.

A Few Words for the Graduates

First, she arranges the tables to form a long rectangle in the center of the conference room. Then she places the orange upholstered chairs around the perimeter, three on each side, two at each end. Ten seats. *That should be enough to hold the group*, she thinks to herself.

Next, she takes a folder of oversized decorative paper out of her carrying case: pink pages printed with bunches of Victorian roses, white sheets with a pattern of pink ribbons and diamond shapes repeated, and some pink and white paper with the words love and hope printed across the top. She carefully places the sheets of paper, one at a time, end-to-end, down the center of the table. Stepping back, she admires her handiwork for a moment. *Looking good*, she thinks to herself.

Finally, she takes twenty photographs from her purse and begins to deal them like playing cards onto the table. One after another, the pictures of the group land face-up on the fancy background papers, until the middle of the table is filled with images of smiling ladies.

Women ranging in age from their early thirties to mid-seventies. Women of every shape and size and lifestyle—married, single, divorced, widowed. Some working, some retired. New mothers, grandmothers and everything in between. All connected by a common disease: breast cancer.

In this small sample of ten breast cancer survivors, there's stage zero to stage four disease. And as a group they have collectively experienced just about every breast cancer treatment in the book—from lumpectomy to bilateral mastectomy to reconstruction and multiple revisions, not to mention, radiation and assorted chemotherapy cocktails. What has bonded them over time is participating in a support group that focuses on the healing power of reading survivor poetry and memoir and then writing the breast cancer experience from their personal points of view.

Seven years, she sighs as she continues fussing with this instant tabletop scrapbook, making sure that the pictures lie straight with equal space between them. Her eyes slowly wander over the snapshots and memories from all those years fill her head.

Here are the ladies wearing matching purple tee shirts, arms linked together as they walk the Survivors' Lap at Relay for Life. Another shot—this time the women are all in pink, performing their original poetry for an audience of survivors at a Living Beyond Breast Cancer networking meeting. In the next photo the women are enjoying a summertime backyard picnic. Here's a good one: all of the ladies standing in a row in front of framed pieces of their writing on display at a Survivor's Day Celebration in Philadelphia. Then there are photographs of birthday celebrations—with lots of presents, colorful balloons and sparkly princess crowns on display. They sure didn't need much of an excuse to get a party going. *Such good times . . . ,* she thinks to herself.

Maybe that's the message for this final meeting of the group, a meeting that just happens to be scheduled during the month of June. A month that's all about graduations: old chapters ending, new chapters beginning. *We have had such good times. And these pictures say it better than words ever could,* she thinks to herself.

But if there's a need for some kind of a graduation speech tonight, it might sound like this:

Tonight is our last formal meeting, ladies, but there's no need for sadness or long faces. In fact, it's just the opposite. We have a lot to smile about! This evening is a celebration of ten incredibly special ladies and seven years of good times. As a group we have combined our collective healing energies and created a loving community, supporting one another through each and every crisis.

And on the bumpy road to recovery, we have all crafted authentic, original, works of art—carefully choosing words and stringing them together to create amazing poems and pieces of memoir describing our experiences. But the best part is that we have shared our creativity with other breast cancer survivors coming up the path behind us. Tonight may not be a classic graduation ceremony—with *Pomp and Circumstance* and caps and gowns and diplomas—but we are truly moving forward. Something special needs to be acknowledged tonight: ladies, we have done such good, healing work together.

She checks her watch. Five minutes to seven. Enough time to do one final thing before the ladies show up at the door. She reaches into her bag and finds a container of small pink plastic gemstones. She sprinkles handfuls of them around the photographs on the table and turns off one bank of overhead lights in the conference room.

From the doorway, in the low light, the tabletop display of photographs is now surrounded by a pale pink glow. It will be the first thing the ladies see when they arrive, moments from now. *Perfect*, she thinks to herself.

It's Not About the Jigsaw Puzzle

It's a puzzle—a 750-piece jigsaw puzzle—spread out on a card table in the far corner of the waiting room, right next to the television. Rumor has it that one of the nurses picked up the jigsaw puzzle at her neighborhood Dollar Store and set it up for the patients the very next day.

It has quickly become the Radiation Oncology waiting room center of attention, competing only occasionally with CNN Headline News and Tyra Banks' latest batch of wacky guests.

When (and if) all of these multicolored puzzle pieces get put together, two whales will breach, side by side, right out of the ocean, silhouetted dramatically against the setting sun. At least, that's what the photo on the jigsaw puzzle box-top promises.

After one month of diligently working this puzzle every morning, along with lots of other cancer survivors in Radiation Oncology, there are moments when I truly have my doubts. *Do you think that all of the pieces are really here? Could some be lost?* (I know that I'm not the only one who has been regularly checking the floor under the table for puzzle pieces that might have gotten away). But maybe that's spoken out of sheer desperation, because for the last week there's been one very noticeable empty spot in the upper left hand corner of the puzzle.

Yes, it's just a Dollar Store jigsaw puzzle (with way too many different shades of 'ocean blueness' going on, if you ask me), but it's starting to feel like so much more than that. Day after day, returning to the Radiation Oncology waiting room for their close encounter with the linear accelerator on the other side of the wall, patients have started hanging out at the card table. In fact, doing the puzzle is becoming a Radiation Oncology waiting room ritual. And like so many CancerLand rituals, it features predictable comments and behaviors.

Here's what happens every morning. The veteran fans of the whale puzzle immediately sit down in one of the four seats at the card table and pick up where the last puzzle solver left off. The straight-edged pieces were clearly the first challenge; they gradually came together to form the puzzle frame. Some folks just enjoy sorting puzzle pieces into piles by color while others focus on one area and fill it in, piece by piece.

Jigsaw puzzle newbies, on the other hand, are more than a little curious about what's going on in the corner, but are still cautious as they approach the card table for the first time. They peek down and typically shake their heads. *Oh, I don't know if I have the patience to do a puzzle with so many pieces in it.* A moment passes. The newbie then tentatively picks up a piece, reaches down and tries to fit it into place. *Hey, does this go here?* Yes, it certainly does and the need to find another puzzle piece that fits (and another and another and another) becomes compelling. Incredibly addictive. The newcomer eventually has no choice but to sit down in one of the empty chairs and get serious.

And so, another new jigsaw puzzle fan is born and joins the team.

Time passes quickly in the waiting room with patients working the puzzle until they hear their names called over the loudspeaker by the nurse, followed by her gentle message: *You can change.*

Sorting pieces. Turning them around. Scanning for shapes. Trial and error, fitting pieces into place and closing gaps. And as they focus on the jigsaw puzzle, the patients stop being strangers and start freely chatting with one another about what's on their minds. While everyone's journey through CancerLand is unique, the need to tell one's story is universal and every bit as compelling as finishing the jigsaw puzzle. And who could be a better audience than someone who is going through a very similar treatment experience?

Heads down and huddled close together over the jigsaw puzzle, with voices slightly above a whisper, the CancerLand conversation flows. One day the topic might be the side effects of radiation. *I'm so itchy. I could just scratch my skin off. What are you using on your skin? I can't find that cream anywhere. I wanted to walk last night but I'm just too tired. You know what I mean?* Or comments about the staff they encounter day after day in Radiation Oncology. *Isn't she the sweetest thing? Do you mind that male tech? Hell, I have no vanity left. Plus he's so professional. My doctor looks so young! I call him Doogie Howser, but not to his face.* And sometimes they look ahead and set intentions for life after radiation ends. *I have four treatments left. I'm going down the shore to celebrate. I'm 83. I'll be happy with just five more years.*

It's just a puzzle on a card table in the corner of the Radiation Oncology waiting room. But it's also a somewhat sacred space where cancer survivors meet and greet one another every morning like old friends and share their stories about getting through treatment. Day after day, small strangely shaped puzzle pieces drop into place, one after another and a colorful picture emerges.

Spirit of Spring

Six brown paper bags, stuffed almost to bursting, sit at the bottom of my basement steps. Long empty of groceries, each bag is filled with another sweet necessity entirely. I inspect these bags every time I pass by—even as I struggle with armloads of laundry on my way to the washing machine. I confess I just can't help myself.

I think about what's inside these bags and it always makes me smile.

These six brown bags have been hiding in my dark unfinished basement since early November. I remember packing them the night of the first fall frost, using sections of the Sunday Inquirer as insulation from the basement dampness. I look at the bags in my basement day after day, week after week, through the cold winter months and think the same thought over and over again: *spring is coming.*

It's all about time, actually. Time passing. Looking forward in time. It's quite intentional on my part. Ritualistic, even. You see, I look at the six brown paper bags and mentally project myself to springtime.

Maybe it's just that time of year right now. All these months of cold, grayness and snow; oh yes, I'm more than a little winter weary. Somehow this brown bag ritual serves me, gets me through. Keeps me upbeat and hopeful, believing that spring will arrive and that I will be here to celebrate the season again.

During the third week of March, these six bags will make the trip up the stairs, out of the dark, into the light, through the house and outside to the turned over and weeded perennial beds in the backyard. For the occasion, I plan to eagerly break out a fresh pair of gloves, slip into my most comfortable stained and well-worn gardening sneakers and (drum roll, please) break open the bags.

By mid-March it's high time to check on the health of my collection of canna bulbs. Some will have rotted, unfortunately, but the majority will be pushing out pale green shoots; ready for planting in my garden. Early spring is the time to get these bulbs back in the ground so that, come July, there will be an amazing field of five foot plus high plants with wide tropical fronds and enough brilliant tomato red colored flowers to stop traffic.

I started this cycle of planting and digging up canna bulbs the summer after my cancer diagnosis. Now (happily) heading into year five of my cancer journey, this bulb-in-the-basement routine is a conscious part of my survivorship strategy. I recommend it highly to my fellow green-thumbed survivors!

Until the buds start peeking out on the trees, until temperatures creep above 32 degrees, keep your heart and spirit as warm as you can. And as we all wait for the official arrival of spring on March 21st, please keep in mind the wise, often quoted words of Hal Borland, "No winter lasts forever, no spring skips its turn. April is a promise that May is bound to keep."

Weeds

Early May and I'm in the backyard, digging up weeds in the garden.

And as I dig around the lilies (still leafing), and the irises (already in bloom: pale yellow, ghostly white and deep purple), I think back five years ago to when this rectangular patch of earth was waist-high in weeds: tall, green, exceptionally healthy weeds.

So healthy in fact that I snipped a bunch of them and delivered them in a plastic bag to the local nursery with a question. "Could these be wildflowers?" I asked hopefully. "I just moved in and I'm not sure yet what's growing out back."

The nursery guy pulled the now somewhat wilted plants out of the bag, one at a time, held them up, and announced in a booming voice, **Weed! Weed! Weed! Weed!** until the bag was empty, much to the amusement of the five master gardeners waiting on line behind me to pay for their plants.

I wanted to disappear. But my humiliation was not complete. Not yet.

"But, hey lady, if you like them," the nursery guy said with a shrug, "just keep watering them and watch them grow."

Yes, I'm in the garden, thinking about the change of seasons and growing things in springtime and weeds that sometimes bloom with brightly colored flowers. And my thoughts turn to cancer, as they often do.

Maybe it's because gardening has become one of my favorite therapies since being diagnosed. Yes, I call it therapy even though a backyard

117

garden is a mixed blessing at best. After all, weeding, planting and maintaining a garden is hard work. Intensely physical and often draining for a middle-aged person, wouldn't you agree? Then there are the other challenges: squirrels that dig up just planted bulbs, rabbits who chew up the tender green shoots just as they push through the soil. On those days, exhausted from the digging and covered head to toe in dirt and grime, (typically with a stubborn fly or two crawling through my hair), I might ask, why bother? What's the point?

Then there are those magical days when a lily opens to the sun and I know it from the moment I first open the porch door and take a step outside. The flower's intense perfume fills the air. Sometimes on a summer afternoon, I can look through the kitchen window and see a butterfly delicately balancing on a bloom in the garden or spot the fluttering of a hummingbird's wings before it zips away. That's when I know that it was all worth it: the hard work and expense, the time and trouble.

When I think about gardening as therapy, I'm reminded of a night so many years ago when a support group member talked about growing flowers in her garden.

She was a fellow breast cancer survivor thrilled by her recovery. Excited to have reached her first goal: five years! She shared with us one way that she was planning to celebrate this momentous occasion: *I've been buying annuals since my diagnosis*, she said. *But this year I am going to start planting perennials again.*

The gardeners in the support group nodded with understanding; (the non-gardeners, not so much). You see, annuals last for only one season. Marigolds, petunias, impatiens; beautiful flowers in vibrant colors, but by summer's end, they're gone, never to return. Perennials, on the other hand, grow back, year after year.

That night in the group some of us learned something new about flowers and gardens. But all of us were schooled in a valuable lesson about hope in CancerLand.

Hope is planting perennials in your garden, believing that you will live to see the flowers bloom next year.

TO ANSWER YOUR QUESTION: WHY I TAKE PICTURES OF FLOWERS . . .

Flowers are not pharmaceuticals.
Flowers are not ports or PICC lines.
pale pink gerbera daisy

Flowers don't need
sentinel node biopsies.
buds closed tight—
squinting eyes in the bright sun

Flowers are never
'one-in-eight.'
delicate dancing yellow iris petals

Flowers are rarely if ever
deleterious mutations.
columbine blooms,
purple and pink wings

Flowers warm my heart.
Flowers fill my senses,
crowding summer's rich color scheme
into my camera lens.
Year after year, flowers heal me—
margins clear and always clean.

Chemo Brain Meets the Inscrutable Relational Database

Last week, almost twelve years to the day after my own cancer diagnosis, I faced up to a daunting challenge that helped me finally make peace with my biggest cancer-related loss to date.

My mind.

If I were writing a cancer memoir, I would call this chapter *Chemo Brain Meets the Inscrutable Relational Database.*

It would go something like this . . .

That day at work, the software trainer treated me like any other student in the class, and that may have been her first mistake.

Standing in the front of the room next to her LCD projector, the trainer began the demonstration, pointing and clicking her way through one screen after another at a breakneck pace, explaining each field and the type of data to be entered in a dull monotone.

Clearly this was a no-nonsense lady with a mission, and her agenda would be accomplished without fail by the scheduled lunch break.

As she spoke, I sat silently next to my computer, a frozen half-smile and less than authentic expression of interest pasted on my face, and tried to take notes on a yellow lined pad. Before long, I was totally lost, not even understanding enough content or process to formulate a coherent question.

The more she lectured, the less I seemed to learn. Minutes ticked by painfully. My discomfort was moving slowly towards full-blown panic; I felt a throbbing headache start up behind my eyes. I furtively looked around the classroom to see if my frustration was mirrored on anybody else's face. Not so much. And that only made me feel worse.

By lunchtime, the other learners had mastered the program and filed out of the training center, leaving me behind—the sole "special needs" student. The "extra help" consisted of the trainer repeating her spiel all over again, starting from the opening screen.

This was about as effective as trying to communicate with an ESL student by simply speaking in a louder voice.

In desperation, I asked the trainer if I could share some feedback on how things were going for me:

I need to tell you why I think I am having so much trouble, I said, *I am a cancer survivor and my treatment included eight rounds of chemotherapy and eight surgeries with general anesthesia. My brain just doesn't work the way it used to. And being middle-aged just makes it worse. Your teaching style doesn't match my learning style. Honestly, I need some accommodations to learn to use this computer program.*

I wish I could tell a story of this software trainer hearing me and adjusting her instructional style accordingly to meet my needs. I wish I could describe a classroom scene where we switched from lecture to hands-on learning with user-friendly cheat sheets in hand to guarantee my success. I'd love to write about such an aha! moment—the lightbulb suddenly turning on and burning brightly over my head. But that would be a lie.

Cancer teaches that I can't change what has happened to my mind and body, (there are no do-overs in CancerLand), but I can try to accept my losses with grace and move forward.

Tutor and Student

"How's it going?" I ask the teenager sitting across from me.

I choose my words carefully before speaking them aloud. Consciously avoid saying *how are you?* Or worse, *how are you feeling?*

He's a kid with cancer getting chemo every three weeks. I'm his assigned English tutor, helping him keep up with his school assignments at home during the "down time" he needs to recover from treatment.

We are working at the family's dining room table that has recently become the student's desk. The dining room is perfectly located for homebound tutoring, mere steps away from the front door. With this arrangement, the tutors don't have far to go once they arrive and the boy's mother can covertly monitor the sessions from the kitchen nearby. There are neat stacks of notebooks and textbooks representing the boy's high school schedule: English, Science, Math and History. A laptop computer is open and waits on standby.

Besides being an English tutor, I'm also a cancer survivor and chemotherapy veteran—experiences that may be much more relevant to this young man right now. More helpful in fact than any advanced American Literature course I aced as an undergraduate.

How weird is this? A teenage boy and a middle-aged woman and here we are, members in the very same club: the Cancer Club. Not by choice, of course, but card-carrying members just the same.

Today our assignment is *Of Mice and Men,* and it's no surprise to me that my student is struggling to remember the details from his reading.

"I think something happens with Lennie and the puppy . . ." he begins, but before long shakes his head in frustration, unable to recall the scene.

"No problem," I say with a smile. "I remember chemobrain." I gently prompt him and together we page through the book to the chapter to tease out the details from the text.

But it's clear that my chemo confession has changed the dynamic between us. My student didn't know that I was in The Cancer Club before and now he does. I feel him looking at me with a different expression on his face: less guarded, more open. Maybe it's because my chemobrain comment leveled the playing field. Forget the teacher/student relationship for the moment. Now we're just two cancer patients chatting together.

Before long we stray from Steinbeck to steroids. "My thoughts jump around like crazy for a few days afterwards," he says. And I am quick to respond, "I know, I know. I couldn't sleep on steroids, so I cleaned out closets instead—lots and lots of closets—and my sock drawer." We debate various ways to mask the metallic taste in your mouth that often comes after chemo. "Have you tried sucking on hard candies?" I ask. "Lemon flavor worked for me."

Our chemo conversation is a tangent, and we'll get back to the rabbits and the American Dream and my lesson plan before long. (all in due time, as the old saying goes). But for now we are fellow travelers in CancerLand, suddenly with so much in common, and a need to share those experiences with one another.

YEARLY CHECK-UP

Twelve years later and not much has changed. Not much. Not really. Starting with the oncologist's grand entrance.

He knocks twice, opens the door and strides into the examining room. His energy speaks volumes (*places to go; patients to see. so many patients; so little time*). I am sitting there, a veteran oncology patient, already changed, perched on the edge of the examining table, a salmon-colored cotton robe wrapped around me.

Welcome to my yearly check-up.

As always, we begin by shaking hands. That's our ritual. Then it's my turn to smile and recite my opening line: *so how's my favorite oncologist?*

Your only oncologist, to the best of my knowledge, Dr. C replies. There he goes—correcting me, reminding me of our running gag about his need for precision, his attention to detail. In CancerLand, Dr. C is a living legend with hundreds of patients' medical records that seem to be stored right in his head. He won't take any notes during the exam and somehow never forgets a date, dosage or chronic complaint. The truth of the matter is that Dr. C dictates his notes on the fly in between patients; sometimes I like to stand outside his office on my way out and listen in.

Regardless, I'll never complain about any quirky personality traits of his. An oncologist who is detail oriented and a bit obsessive is a *good* thing, don't you think?

Any lumps, bumps or bruises? Dr. C asks, moving briskly into Act One: The Physical Exam. I lie flat on my back. He modestly opens the gown, uncovering one side at a time, keeping the opposite side hidden, and presses the tips of his fingers in a circular pattern. Then he says the word I've been patiently waiting for (*perfect*) as he finishes with the left side and moves around the table to begin his exam of the right. Twelve years of exams later and like an addict hungry for a fix, I inhale the word (*perfect*), and savor how good it feels (*I'm okay, I'm okay*).

But honestly, is this ironic, or what? After all, there might be a short list of politically (and clinically) correct terms that could be used to describe my post-treatment upper body (*altered? revised? reconstructed?*) But perfect? Hardly.

Does this doctor who deals with so many breast cancer survivors know the impact of his word choice? Or is "perfect" the word this particular oncologist has decided to use with his patients to indicate that there's no sign of disease? All I know is that perfect is a lovely word, and I can't wait to hear him say it.

The exam comes to a predictable conclusion with light banter about our personal lives and those acquaintances we have in common, and that's when I suddenly think of a word that I want to add to our yearly check-up script.

So, tell me, Alysa, Dr. C asks, moving towards the door, ready to conclude the exam. *Overall, how was your year?*

I'm ready with the perfect answer.

Unremarkable, I say, *my year was unremarkable.* And I see the doctor cock his head with interest. I have never used this term in our conversations before. Over the years, he has, of course. To describe my CAT scans, bloodwork and Breast MRI results. To report that everything is normal, that there is nothing out of the ordinary.

An unremarkable year, I repeat. *No surgeries. I'm hoping that next year turns out to be another unremarkable year. Unremarkable totally works for me.*

It certainly does. And now that I've said it out loud, this is an intention I plan to keep. Day by day, I need to hold it close until I'm in this examining room again, twelve months from today for my next yearly check-up.

A disease-free reality; in my mind that's the most remarkable thing I can imagine.

Something Good

Something good. The first time I tried it, and it worked, no one was more surprised than me.

Let me explain:

Over the summer I struggled with a bad case of the blues: long weeks of low energy and negative thoughts, little or no enthusiasm to make plans with other people. Way too much time spent sitting alone and numb in front of the TV, hypnotized by old movies and summer reruns.

How weird to feel so down, so listless, so unmotivated and not know the reason why. I couldn't blame my ongoing sadness on any recent crisis in my life. Or on one of those *I'm-sorry-I-have-some-bad-news-for-you* phone calls from an onco-doc. And it certainly wasn't a nasty side effect of any new pharmaceutical in my medicine cabinet.

So I analyzed and ultimately rationalized my situation this way: *can't mood swings happen to the best of us, whether or not we are in—or outside of CancerLand?* This psychological low point just *was*—and clearly in my life right now for no particular reason I could fathom. But the truth was, I hated feeling this way. I wanted the 'old me' back.

How could I short-circuit my blue mood and put a smile back on my face?

Then I remembered the idea of setting positive intentions. Maybe I read about it in one of those books I find myself constantly skimming in the self-help section at Barnes & Noble. (You know the ones I'm talking about—they have catchy, italicized subtitles with lots of exclamation points—*Take control of your life now!!!*). Maybe I heard about it on *Oprah* or *Dr. Phil.* All I know is that I was at a point where I had nothing to lose and everything to gain, so I did it: I started setting positive intentions.

Once I made up my mind to try it, beginning the process was incredibly easy. Driving to work the next morning, I picked a positive thought (*something good will happen today*), and repeated it silently to myself over and over again until I pulled into the parking lot.

The next step would be more of a challenge. I had to wait and see what my first *something good* would turn out to be.

That night there it was, *something good* sitting in my mailbox, tucked neatly between the bills and Home Depot circulars: a handmade thank you card from a fellow cancer survivor. She wrote, *how can I ever thank you for all you've done for me and all you've been for me in some of my darkest hours?* Wow! I was touched by her kind words and totally freaked out by her incredible timing.

The next morning *something good* turned out to be a parade of geese stopping traffic to walk across a busy suburban side street to reach the pond on the other side of the road. This updated version of *Make Way for Ducklings* immediately put a big smile on my face.

On Saturday afternoon *something good* was my three year old neighbor Margo running into my yard with her child-sized toy rake in hand to help me clean up the first fall leaves of the season. After raking diligently for a few minutes, Margo bent over and picked up a few acorns from the ground.

She held them out to me in the palm of her hand and announced proudly, "Coconuts for you."

Forever the teacher, I gently corrected her. "Those are actually acorns, Margo."

"No, coconuts," she insisted.

What is the name of a round object that falls from a tree that has a hard outside shell? Hmmmmmm. I tried to see the world through her three-year old eyes and couldn't help but smile.

It is all how you look at it, isn't it?

Another day *something good* was the e-mail I got from the public library announcing that a *New York Times* bestseller that I had put on reserve over a month ago was now waiting for me to pick it up.

Before long *something good* was peeking through the kitchen window at the morning glories climbing the patio fence, blossoms wide open in shades of pale blue and hot pink at 6:30 a.m.

Something good was also silently watching a pair of tiger swallowtails lazily explore purple flowers blooming on the backyard butterfly bush.

No doubt about it. *Something good* was working wonderfully well for me, so I continued the experiment. Day after day, during my daily commute, I diligently repeated to myself the same positive intention. By dinnertime I reviewed the day's events to pick out *something good* that had happened. Soon it became obvious that this process created a marvelous tension, powerful enough to lift my spirits for most of the day.

Finally, I had to ask, did setting the positive intention actually make *something good* happen? Was I in fact drawing happiness and joy towards me like a magnet? Or did this process just supply the attitude adjustment, helping me to focus on the many small and precious moments that can be uplifting, only if we are properly "tuned in" to experience them?

Was it the chicken or the egg? In the end, does it matter?

Today *something good* is completing this piece and sharing it with all of you.

SPLENDIDLY IMPERFECT 50/50

Last time I checked, cancer is *not* a comedy. No way. No how. Not even close. Maybe that's why I was so disturbed by the movie trailer for *50/50* when it first appeared on TV last year.

For some unknown reason, they seemed to be marketing this cancer movie as a comedy. Seriously. Even though there's not much plot-wise to put a smile on anyone's face: a man in his late twenties tries to cope with treatment for a malignant tumor in his spine.

(Wait. Don't laugh yet. There's more . . .)

The patient's dire diagnosis translates into multiple rounds of chemotherapy followed by high-risk surgery. Along the way, his artist/ girlfriend cheats on him, his mother tries to "smother love" the cancer right out of him and his best friend uses a head newly bald from chemo as a cool way to meet girls in bars and bookstores. Good times!

The *50/50* movie trailer made me so mad that I even started complaining about it to a friend who happens to be a fellow cancer survivor.

"Maybe the movie's not *funny-ha-ha*," said my friend. "Maybe it's more *funny-ironic*. We should definitely go check it out."

"I don't know about that . . ." I responded. Then my friend suggested an alternate theory.

"Maybe they're calling *50/50* a comedy just to sell movie tickets . . ." she said, her voice trailing off.

What was left unspoken was this: who in their right mind would make a *serious* movie about cancer and actually expect people to queue up and pay the current high price of a movie ticket to see it as *entertainment?*

Who, indeed? All I can say is that when *50/50* first hit the theatres last year, I was torn, feeling a real "push-pull": *wanting* to see the movie because of the subject matter, *avoiding* seeing the movie because of the subject matter. Do you know what I mean?

Fast forward to now. *50/50* is out on DVD, as well as available on demand. Let the record show that today I surrendered without much of a fight to watch the movie in the privacy of my own living room.

And just as I suspected, *50/50* is definitely NOT a comedy; (I didn't laugh at all; in fact I actually cried my way through half a box of Kleenex before the credits rolled). But that's just fine with me because cancer is *not* a comedy. Instead, *50/50 is* a wonderful film that focuses in a meaningful way on the cancer patient experience.

The movie shares moments—intense moments—that will ring true to many CancerLand veterans. Our hero gets the bad news sitting in his doctor's office and the image on the screen immediately goes out of focus and the audio fades away. What a powerful way to depict the shock of a cancer diagnosis!

His doctor stays in a cold, clinical mode as he speaks with his patient about the treatment plan for his cancer. And his response to his patient's deer-in-the-headlights expression is to immediately offer him the services of capable psychologists and social workers on staff.

Our newly diagnosed hero immediately makes an appointment to get some of that prescribed emotional support and discovers that he is patient #3 for a graduate student completing her dissertation. She quotes the psychosocial literature admirably, but is unable to be present and offer much comfort to a patient who is unnerved by life and death concerns, beyond patting his arm mechanically (*there, there, this must be difficult for you . . .*) as she has been very well trained to do.

Chemotherapy in the film is depicted as a social experience fueled by shared patient anger as well as home-baked cookies laced with marijuana. The newbie learns the ropes from two older cancer patients sitting in nearby barcaloungers who introduce themselves with the stage and location of their cancers. The instant intimacy among cancer patients is good medicine of another sort entirely, and our hero soon enjoys the benefits of connecting with fellow travelers on the road to recovery.

Caregivers try. They really do. But the truth is obvious—it's not easy supporting a cancer patient who is going through the rigors of treatment. *50/50* introduces us to a girlfriend who admits she would rather wait for hours in the car than accompany her boyfriend into the Chemo Lounge. (*I need to keep my energy separate from that*), and to a best friend who secretly reads books in the bathroom with titles like *How to Talk to a Cancer Patient* and thoughtfully dog ears the best parts. The cancer patient's mother confesses that she attends a support group for relatives to cope with her son's health crisis. The details ring true because no doubt they *are* true; the screenplay was written by a cancer survivor.

Unlike various other cancer-themed movies that have played on the big and small screen over the years, these characters are based on real people and they act in believable ways. They live and breathe on the screen. They say the wrong thing at the wrong time. They mean well. They really do. But they are just like the rest of us—flawed, splendidly imperfect human beings trying to cope in the face of a health crisis.

If there is any humor in *50/50* it's the chuckle of recognition, of seeing yourself, of seeing people you know and love being portrayed by famous actors in someone else's cancer story. If you have spent any time at all in CancerLand, the situations and the behaviors on the screen will speak to you and remind you of parts of your own journey through treatment.

And if you're like me, watching *50/50* might move you to play back the mental movie of your own experience, help you acknowledge that you did the best that you could at the time, help you forgive yourself first and then everyone in your inner circle second. After all that, you just might sigh loudly and have a good cry. Not to worry; that's the great thing about catharsis—it's all good . . .

Cancer survivors, caregivers, doctors, nurses and social workers interacting with cancer patients, please add *50/50* to your "must see" list and see if you don't agree with me.

One Good Thing About My Yearly Mammogram

I'm in
and out of
there, I swear,
in the blink of an
eye. Moving at warp
speed, clothes peeled to
the waist in seconds flat.
Motion lines blur, tremble
on either side of me. I fight
off demons that recur, mute
their evil chatter (*we found it
once, we'll find it again*). Steal
a quick glance down at my
watch. It's official: I'm in
and out and on my way,
I'd say in maybe *half*
the time it takes
everybody else.

Sometimes I Almost Forget

Sometimes a day goes by, my cancer survivor buddy Lydia says wistfully, *a whole day and I don't think about it once. Not once! I can almost forget I* had *cancer, you know what I mean?* And she says those words with this incredulous expression on her face, shaking her head from side to side as if to say, *can you believe it? can you imagine? is such a thing actually possible?*

I don't know if in fact I do know what she means. But I listen and try on that feeling for size, to see how it fits.

Hours later I am sitting on my yoga mat, legs crisscrossed under me, listening to the teacher direct the class from the front of the room. She models our next posture—a seated twist—while she speaks the directions aloud to us in her gentle voice: . . . *lift both your arms to the side . . . take a deep breath . . . extend from the waist . . . as you exhale, reach with your right arm for your left knee, twist at the waist and look over your left shoulder.*

I listen to the George Winston piano CD playing in the background. I breathe deeply. I direct my cancer-treated, middle-aged body to move. At that moment, the yoga teacher adds a postscript to her directions. What I refer to as the Yoga Blessing: *if it's available to you,* she says. Words that in my humble opinion ought to be part of life outside the yoga studio, part of life "off the mat" if you will: The Yoga Blessing is a caveat that encourages practice, while at the same time discourages competition and comparison with others. *If it's available to you . . .* I love it! Ultimately this is a caution against performing at a level that you may not be ready for. Not now. Not yet.

That's the moment when I feel a sharp stabbing pain in the area below my right shoulder blade—the place where a muscle was removed by a plastic surgeon ten years ago to reconstruct my right breast. My gasp must be audible because the yoga teacher immediately looks in my direction and asks calmly, *are you okay? Pain during yoga class is not okay. Listen to your body.*

Good advice. I hear my body's protest loud and clear and move tentatively into the child's pose, head down, face to the mat. I surrender to the pain that has turned into a spasm across my back and breathe into it while soothing music continues to play in the background.

As I wait for the pain to subside, I play back in my head my friend's comments from earlier in the day (*I can almost forget I had cancer),* and hear a voice in my head say, *that's just not available to you yet.*

But what a lovely thought . . .

The Box

I have a box. It says breast cancer on the lid.
I opened the box because 1. I had no choice.
2. They all told me to. 3. Maybe I wanted to
test myself to see if I was strong enough to
pry the lid off, peer into the darkness,
then slam the box shut. All by myself.
Yes I am. Yes I can. Yes I did.

ACKNOWLEDGMENTS

I'm a born storyteller, so once I landed in CancerLand, there was a wide writing territory to explore. But no one makes this journey alone. Here are some of the people who helped me find my way—guiding me towards recovery (and publication), talking me down from the ledge as I moved from point A to point B:

Warmest thanks to the ladies of Bosom Buddies and Pink Ribbon Poetry, who were my first audiences and most enthusiastic cheerleaders.

John Fox introduced me to poetry therapy in one unforgettable workshop and Dr. Sherry Reiter coached me on the long and winding road to certification as a poetry therapist. Their collective feedback that my stories were worth telling motivated me to find new ways to serve fellow cancer survivors.

I am beholden to Colleen Carey Merrell, the oncology nurse who patiently listened to my CancerLand stories, and helped me channel my anger into supporting other breast cancer patients.

Thank you many times over to Drs. Maurice Cairoli, Eric Miller and Angela Veloudios. These three gifted healers shared a precious gift with me; the insight that, in CancerLand, every day is Thanksgiving.

Everybody needs an angel (or two) in life and mine is Amy Grillo from Living Beyond Breast Cancer. Without her support and legendary attention to detail, Writing the Journey would be just another idea on a whiteboard. Thank you, Amy, for believing in me and for helping me fill all the seats around the library's conference table.

Reading cancer memoirs and poetry moved me to try and tell my story too. These are some of the CancerLand authors and poets whose books fill my shelves, whose collective talent humbles me, whose words continue to inspire my own: Kelly Corrigan, Julia Darling, Barbara Delinsky, Caryn Mirriam Goldberg, Laurie Kingston, Alicia Ostriker, Katherine Russell Rich, Dan Shapiro, Suzanne, Strempek Shea, Anne Silver and Joyce Wadler.

I will be forever grateful to my editors Maggie Hampshire and Carolyn Vachani at OncoLink for answering my emails, for a decade of unwavering support (*Love it! Love it! Love it!*) and for one especially encouraging message (*you should write a book—get on that!*)

First time authors definitely need a muse that sits right next to the keyboard, and mine is a beautiful brown striped tabby, appropriately named Hope.

Finally, special thanks to Chuck and Phyllis for being no more than two rings away, and for laughing at all the punchlines.

Alysa Cummings is a certified poetry therapist and breast cancer survivor who believes in the healing power of writing. *Greetings in CancerLand* features her favorite anecdotes and poems describing the cancer experience. Many of these pieces have appeared previously, from 2002-2012 as online projects and blog postings on the OncoLink website (www.oncolink.org) where Alysa has been named Poet-in-Residence. When Alysa is not writing, she is busy leading writing workshops in New Jersey—helping other cancer survivors tell their CancerLand stories. This is her first book.

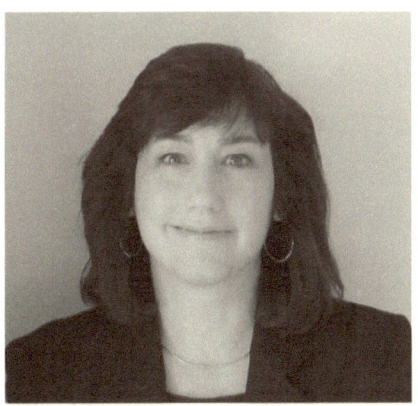